BASIC HEALTH PUBLICATIONS USER'S GUIDE

TO
ENERGY-BOOSTING SUPPLEMENTS

Discover the Best
Supplements for Safely
Enhancing Your
Energy Levels.

RONALD HUNNINGHAKE, M.D.,
AND MELISSA LYNN BLOCK
JACK CHALLEM Series Editor

The information contained in this book is based upon the research and personal and professional experiences of the authors. It is not intended as a substitute for consulting with your physician or other healthcare provider. Any attempt to diagnose and treat an illness should be done under the direction of a healthcare professional.

The publisher does not advocate the use of any particular healthcare protocol but believes the information in this book should be available to the public. The publisher and authors are not responsible for any adverse effects or consequences resulting from the use of the suggestions, preparations, or procedures discussed in this book. Should the reader have any questions concerning the appropriateness of any procedures or preparations mentioned, the authors and the publisher strongly suggest consulting a professional healthcare advisor.

Series Editor: Jack Challem
Editor: Susan Andrews
Typesetter: Gary A. Rosenberg
Series Cover Designer: Mike Stromberg

Basic Health Publications User's Guides are published by Basic Health Publications, Inc.

ISBN: 978-1-59120-176-2 (Pbk.)
ISBN: 978-1-68162-852-3 (Hardcover)

CONTENTS

INTRODUCTION

I, Ronald Hunninghake, have a confession to make: I'm a doctor, writing a book about energy . . . and I used to suffer terribly from fatigue! I did not have chronic fatigue syndrome, I was not depressed, and I had no serious illnesses, such as diabetes. I enjoyed my work. My wife and family were wonderful. I slept well (though probably not enough). I walked every day and kept my weight down. In spite of all this, I was pooped!

I could make it through the day all right, but only after a cappuccino jump-start in the morning, a noon nap, and several diet colas in the afternoon. Even then, I would typically experience a "brown-out" between two and three o'clock each day—my eyes heavy, my facial expression drooping, and my attention drifting into semiconscious drowsiness. It wasn't unusual for a patient to jolt me back to reality with a sharp "Doctor . . . doctor! Are you okay?"

No, I wasn't okay. Something was wrong that I didn't see and couldn't understand. I was so immersed in my fatigue, I made the mistake of assuming everyone felt tired. In a sense, I had "adapted" to my fatigue. Looking back, I now know that I was very low in energy, and I didn't know how to correct the situation.

Though not overweight, I was often hungry, and usually for the wrong things. If there were something sugary that I could get my hands on, I would go for that. I knew I needed more energy and was looking for some way to "infuse" it into my body.

Quick calories gave me a quick burst of energy, like a roller coaster making it to the top of a steep climb. Then, my blood sugar would plummet, and I would often feel things going fuzzy, as though I were going to black out.

In a very real sense, these were moments when I had "run out of gas." Filling the tank over and over again with sugary foods wasn't working. Indeed, for many of my patients, this approach to fatigue was leading to weight gain in their abdominal area. This central obesity—coupled with a tendency for high blood pressure, high cholesterol and blood lipids, and borderline blood sugar readings—form an ominous medical constellation that over a third of Americans now face: Syndrome X, also known as "metabolic syndrome." This syndrome leads directly to the fastest-growing disease in America today: type 2 diabetes. The onset of type 2 diabetes is often heralded by severe fatigue.

In fact, *many* medical conditions are associated with fatigue. That's why people often say they are "sick and tired" of frustrating life situations. They are definitely tired, and often sick. And why does tiredness often precede diabetes and many other serious illnesses? *It's because the key cellular nutrients needed to run the biochemistry of energy production are depleted.*

Could it be that overeating is an attempt to get these needed nutrients? When the basic understanding of cellular energy production is missing, humans will forage blindly in their attempt to fill in this gap. Obesity (another major cause of fatigue and illness) may be the result of a misdirected attempt to correct cellular malnutrition.

Feeding the Fire

The purpose of this book is to introduce you to a basic understanding of bioenergetics. "Bio" is life. "Energetics" is energy. Bioenergetics is the study of the energy of life. This is basic biochemistry 101. Unfortunately, biochemistry is usually locked up in textbooks, where sleepy-eyed students study it for the purpose of passing a test. Knowing how energy is created at the cellular level and how to feed those processes helps us pass the most important test: how we live our day-to-day lives.

Dr. Hugh Riordan, the founder of the center where I have practiced for the past two decades, offered this definition of health: *Health is having the reserves to do what you need to do and want to do with **energy** and enthusiasm.* This is a functional definition. Health is a doing thing. One cannot do without energy! (And enthusiasm is energy with an attitude!) The scientist who discovered vitamin C, Albert Szent-Györgyi, referred to energy as the "currency" of life. Without energy, you have nothing to spend!

I began this introduction by admitting my helplessness in the face of unrelenting fatigue. That was years ago, when I was "energy-ignorant." Through a better understanding of bioenergetics, I was able to overcome my own tiredness and lethargy. I now know that there are ways to revive and enliven the bioenergetic system. I know, because I have helped many chronically tired patients to regain their energy and to become "colearners" in the process.

Dr. Riordan coined this term. Colearners are patients who take an active role in the discovery of the actual underlying causes of their illness. Colearners are partners with health professionals. I invite you to become a colearner with my coauthor, Melissa Block, and me. We wrote this book to help you conquer fatigue and enjoy a more energetic life.

As a colearner, you will better understand how cellular energy—a kind of "cellular fire"—is created and sustained. Like any fire, if it is fed poorly selected fuel (see Chapter 2), it will become weak. If the kindling is wet (see Chapter 3) it will not ignite properly. If care is not taken to tend to the sparks flying off the blaze (see Chapter 4), damage to the surrounding cellular environment can ensue. By knowing which kinds of wood to use, you can make your fire burn in a slower and more sustained fashion (see Chapter 5) or faster and hotter (see Chapter 6). There are ways to stoke your fire's reserves as well (see Chapter 7).

We use the analogy of building a fire very purposefully here. Those of you who camp or own a wood fireplace know that building a fire is both a skill and an art form! Every fire is unique, but predictable. If you take care and make good choices, your fire will rise up into a wondrous thing of beauty, bringing light, warmth, and utility to your experience. If you approach your fire in a haphazard fashion, or are ignorant of what constitutes a healthy fire, you will be disappointed . . . and probably end up with a lot of smoke!

Like this fire, cellular energy is your creation. If you take it for granted and ignore the basics of bioenergetics, then you can predict the outcome you will experience: fatigue!

Should you take ownership of your cellular fire, feed it properly, tend to it carefully, stoke it, and learn the basics of maintaining it, you will be rewarded with an experience of great personal empowerment. You will overcome chronic fatigue and replace it with a sustainable experience of energy and hope.

This book will be your cellular fire-building guide!

CHAPTER 1

How Your Body Makes Energy

Long ago, early humans figured out how to make fire. This knowledge gave us greater adaptability and a wider range of choices. Once limited to temperate climates, humans were capable of migrating to colder regions of the earth. Fire meant cooked food, warmer shelters, and greater safety from wild animals.

In many ways, the discovery of fire was the beginning of civilization. Fire became the center of tribal culture. Fire keeping may have been the first human profession! Fire metaphors are tightly woven into our language: hearts on fire with passion, the fire in the belly, the burning desire for knowledge, fear of getting "burned."

Fire remains a dramatic force in human life today. Forest fires and fires in homes and businesses can bring great destruction and fear. But what could be more comforting than a fire in the fireplace or a campfire on a cool night?

Like most natural forces, fire is both good and bad. This book is about another kind of natural fire that can be both good and bad. This is an inner, unseen fire, burning every second of your life, the source of all life and all biological activity. Without it, you would be extinguished.

This fire takes place within cells, the basis of all life on this planet. Cells breathe, metabolize, live, grow, divide, and replicate based on life processes that depend on energy. Life depends on energy. And energy is fire!

The Fire of Metabolism

At the level of the cells in your body, a kind of fire is burning, too. This "fire"—made in the metabolic machinery of each cell, known as the *mitochondria*—creates heat and energy. Our warm-bloodedness and the physical energy that enables us to do, feel, and be so much originates in these microscopic fires that burn in almost every cell in our bodies.

Just as fire can be either a blessing or a curse, so, too, is the fire of metabolism. If fed and managed properly, and kept contained, this fire supports optimum energy for us to do what we need to do in our lives. If mismanaged with inappropriate fuel sources, or if there are inadequate barriers to keeping the metabolic "fire" from burning out of control, the fire that sustains us can come back to injure us.

This book is about managing the fires that create cellular energy in your body—and about what can go wrong if those fires aren't properly contained or supported. Appropriate diet, supplements, and lifestyle habits like regular exercise and stress reduction all play a role in maintaining and taming the metabolic fires inside you, and this is what you'll learn about in the pages of this book.

The Energy Spectrum

Elite endurance athletes could practically be considered their own species, separated from the rest of us humans by their ability to run, or swim, or cycle, or do a combination of these things, for miles and miles—*fast*.

And, even more unbelievably, doing so feels good to them. Their muscles, hearts, and respiratory systems are far more efficient than those of the average person. If they miss a day, or are injured and miss a few weeks, they don't feel like themselves. Something about their bodies makes these rare individuals want to go and go and go—the human equivalents of the Energizer Bunny.

At the other extreme are people who have genetic disorders that hamper the capacity of their bodies to make adequate energy: *mitochondrial myopathies*, which bring about intense and constant fatigue. Scientific studies show that flaws in their muscle-cell DNA render cellular energy production markedly inefficient.

There are many factors that create the difference between the elite athlete and the mitochondrial myopathy patient, including the pumping strength of the heart, the ability of the respiratory system to take in adequate oxygen and blow off enough carbon dioxide, and the amount of fuel (glucose, the simplest form of sugar) that can be stored in the liver.

But the factor we'll focus on here is differences between the muscle cells of the former—which are far more efficient at producing lots of energy over long periods of time—and the latter. The process of *metabolism*, where fuel is burned in the cells to produce energy, runs more smoothly and efficiently in the athlete, making more energy to fuel the body's efforts. (Even the average Joe who prefers couch-sitting to running marathons has far more efficient cellular metabolism than the unfortunate person with mitochondrial myopathy.)

To set the stage for learning about energy nutrients, let's look specifically at the metabolic process: how the "fires" of metabolism release the energy in food as energy in our bodies.

Vitamins and other substances found in foods play a major role in this process. When you see how most of the several trillion cells in your body create their own supply of energy, you'll better understand how the various nutrients and dietary changes we recommend in the rest of this book work to promote improved energy production *at the level of individual cells*—and how this adds up to improvements in energy levels that you can feel.

The Mystery and Magic of Energy

In traditional Chinese medicine (TCM) and the ancient Indian medical art called Ayurveda, energy is at the crux of disease, diagnosis, and treatment. TCM has mapped complex networks of *meridians*, or energy channels, along which acupuncture needles are specifically placed to direct or redirect the flow of energy, or *qi* (also spelled *chi*). Foods, medical therapies, and lifestyle choices are believed to carry specific energies, either *yin* or *yang*, and the balance of those energies has a lot to do with one's state of health.

In Ayurveda, each person's constitution is composed of a combination of three *doshas*, each of which has physical, emotional, and energetic characteristics. Moving a person toward health involves foods, bodywork, and other therapies designed to adjust the balance of the doshas in the body.

Yoga, tai chi, chi kung, and other forms of "enlightened exercise" are all about moving energy inside the body in ways that increase vitality and defuse stress. (This is addressed in more detail in Chapter 8.)

The one thing all of these medical schools of thought and body therapies have in common: *they work.* They heal. If you truly engage yourself in their practice, and become an active participant—colearner—who uses his or her mind and will to adjust the energies that flow within your body, you will feel and function better. Such practices modulate the metabolic fires, helping to keep them high enough to yield optimum energy, but not high enough to do damage.

Sometimes, this kind of whole-body energy work may not be enough to renew energy. If you are fatigued and having trouble keeping up with your life, some nutritional "tweaking" may be needed to nourish your body at the cellular level. This is especially likely to be true if you don't eat an ideal diet rich in vegetables, whole grains, fruits, fish, nuts, and seeds; and if you live a typically fast-paced, energy-draining lifestyle.

It's humbling to acknowledge that the energy that powers our bodies is inextricably linked to the energy that makes trees grow, makes the earth turn, and moves oceans and mountains. It's inspiring to recognize that we can, to some extent, control the flow of that energy, and enrich its availability within our bodies at the cellular level.

The energy that powers your body originates in individual cells, which need a certain amount of energy to do their jobs in the body. And in the cells of humans and animals, that energy is brought out within tiny cellular "engines" called *mitochondria*.

The Mighty Mitochondria

The mitochondria is the part of the cell that is charged with the important job of producing energy to fuel the various processes that maintain it. There are around 2,500 mitochondria in almost every body cell—microscopic "furnaces," if you like. Within these oval-shaped organelles are numerous enzymes. These enzymes act on *glucose*, the simplest breakdown form of carbohydrates in the diet, to make potential energy in the form of a substance called ATP (adenosine triphosphate). When ATP is transformed into ADP, that energy—the heat from the "fire"—is liberated to fuel the work of the cell.

> **Enzyme**
> *A protein produced by living cells that promotes or otherwise influences biochemical reactions.*

Cell Metabolism (Bioenergetics) Made Simple

When you eat a meal, it is broken down into its simplest components in the digestive tract. Carbohydrates are broken down into glucose; fats, into fatty acids; and proteins, into amino acids. These substances pass through the walls of the small intestine into large blood vessels. From there, large blood vessels branch off into ever-smaller vessels, until they become hair-thin *capillaries*. Through the one-cell-layer-thick walls of these capillaries, glucose, fatty acids, and amino acids move through the outer membranes of individual cells. (The hormone insulin is required for glucose to make this passage; insulin resistance, a prediabetic condition, is notorious for robbing the body of energy, because the ability of the body cells to move glucose into the cells decreases.)

Bioenergetics
A general term that describes the sum total of energy-producing processes in living cells.

Amino acids become building blocks for the creation and repair of enzymes and cellular structures. Fatty acids can be used as fuel in the mitochondria, but it first has to be transformed into glucose through a process called *beta-oxidation*—more on this later in the chapter.

Glucose passes right into the mitochondria, where it is dismantled by enzymes in two different processes: the first is called *glycolysis*, and the second is called the *Krebs cycle*.

Glycolysis

Glycolysis (gly-KOH-luh-sis) is the first step in the three-step process that turns glucose into energy. It doesn't require oxygen, so it's also referred to as *anaerobic* (without oxygen) metabolism. It transforms glucose into a substance called *pyruvate*, and creates two ATP—remember, that's the "fuel" used by the cell—in the process. Pyruvate is the raw material—the breakdown product of glucose—that is transformed by other enzymes into a substance called *acetyl coA*.

When the body is at rest, or when it's exerting itself in a moderate fashion, acetyl coA then passes into the Krebs cycle, part two of the three-part process that turns glucose into energy. If the body is in vigorous motion, under undue stress, or not producing energy efficiently, it may not smoothly shift pyruvate into the Krebs cycle.

Imagine a sprinter dashing out of the starting blocks. Her muscles require lots of energy, quickly. For that energy, her body will rely upon glycolysis, because it can produce energy rapidly—a quick-starting, high-flaring fire.

The Krebs cycle chugs along fine as long as energy requirements remain more or less fixed. When you're at rest or moderately exerting yourself, the fire of metabolism burns at a low level, making energy steadily without rapidly depleting your fuel reserves.

When energy needs increase dramatically and quickly, muscle cells revert to glycolysis for most of the energy needed. Consider it fast-food energy: you're hungry *now*, so you pull into the drive-through and get substandard fare that fills your belly but doesn't fortify you for the long haul.

Glycolysis is very inefficient compared with the Krebs cycle. The Krebs cycle yields from twenty to thirty-six ATP per molecule of glucose; glycolysis only ekes out two ATP per glucose. Another problem: when the body relies heavily on glycolysis, pyruvate begins to accumulate. The excess is transformed into *lactic acid,* which lowers muscular pH and can lead to fatigue, muscle cramps, and general lack of endurance.

Imagine yourself jogging on the treadmill. You can do six miles per hour without much trouble, and you can maintain that pace for a half hour or more. But if you crank the speed up to seven miles per hour, your breathing gets labored and your leg muscles start to burn within five minutes. At six miles per hour, your body can get oxygen to the cells at a rate adequate to maintain the Krebs cycle, but at seven miles per hour, your cells start to rely on glycolysis. Lactic acid starts to accumulate in your muscles, hence "the burn" we were once told to go for while exercising. The rate at which your muscles require energy is too rapid for the Krebs cycle and its partner, the *electron transport chain*, to kick in.

Remember our friend with the mitochondrial myopathy? Her muscle cells are missing or low on some of the "equipment" required to push pyruvate into the Krebs cycle. Her muscles rely primarily upon glycolysis for energy production. Her fires burn high and fast, but she quickly runs out of fuel. As a result, she has little endurance and feels tired much of the time.

Natural therapies that supply cells with extra nutrients required for the Krebs cycle can aid individuals with these rare genetic conditions. There's more about this in chapters to come.

The Krebs Cycle and the Electron Transport Chain

Although this might sound like the name of a funk band, it actually describes the two remaining processes that occur in your cells to release energy from glucose so that it can be put to work inside those cells.

Basically, the Krebs cycle involves the sequential extraction of electrons from what's left of the glucose molecule following glycolysis. With each extraction, energy is released, and by the end of the cycle, glucose has become carbon dioxide, the waste product of metabolism.

The electrons that are pulled off of glucose, which is a six-carbon molecule that happens to contain lots of electrons, are then shuttled out to the mitochondrial membrane by specialized enzymes. Those electrons are then "accepted" by oxygen molecules in the mitochondrial membrane. Finally, the oxygen plus the electron is transformed into water.

The electron transport chain is where the energy created during the dismantling of glucose is packaged as ATP—remember, that's between twenty and thirty-six ATP per glucose molecule. Once formed, ATP drifts to the places in the cell where work needs to be done and is broken apart into ADP (adenosine diphosphate) and a free phosphate (P), thereby releasing its energy. The ADP and P are then available to be made into another ATP as the cycle continues.

Every turn of the Krebs cycle and the production of energy by the electron transport chain requires oxygen. It also requires nutrients—a lot of nutrients, including vitamin B_1 (thiamine), vitamin B_2 (riboflavin), and vitamin B_3 (niacin), all of which act as *coenzymes* that keep the enzymatic machinery of metabolism in motion. Cellular metabolism also requires coenzyme Q_{10}, alpha-lipoic acid (a nutrient made in the body), pantothenic acid (another nutrient in the B-vitamin class), and several minerals and amino acids.

> Scientists estimate that as we age, the efficiency and quantity of our mitochondria decrease; cells are operating at only one-half to one-quarter the energy supply we have in youth.

Beta-Oxidation

Your body constantly burns fats in your cells to create the fires of energy production, but first it has to turn them into acetyl coA—the substance that enters the Krebs cycle—in the mitochondria through a process called *beta-oxidation*. Once that has happened, the rest of the cycle follows, just as it does with carbohydrates.

Some fatty acids also require the support of a substance called *carnitine* to pass through the cell wall to be turned into glucose and burned for energy. The carnitine gets the fuel to where it can be burned by the metabolic fires. Carnitine is addressed in detail in Chapter 5.

Oxidative Metabolism Catch-22

If you are knowledgeable about diet and health, you probably recognize the word *oxidation* as something that isn't good for the body. Oxidation is another word for the production of free radicals—reactive free electrons that, when not "quenched" by antioxidants, can damage fats, proteins, and genetic material (DNA and RNA). If you know that much, you probably also know that free radicals have been implicated as a causative factor in heart disease, Alzheimer's disease, cancer, and many other conditions.

Free radicals are produced abundantly during oxidative metabolism. You might think of them as smoke from the metabolic fires. Free radicals are the carriers of energy through the complex Krebs cycle and electron transport chain. Some free radicals "leak" out of the biochemical reactions that maintain cellular energy—particularly when bioenergetics become less efficient.

Free radicals may also have something to do with low energy—not just because of the diseases for which they can set the stage. Free radicals that leak from bioenergetic processes can damage genetic material within the mitochondria, further decreasing its efficiency. They can spark oxidative chain reactions that eventually lead to cellular dysfunction and demise.

We're only as healthy as the cells that comprise our organs, and as the organs that make up our body systems, and so the first link in the chain of excellent health and high energy is to try to nourish each of our cells the best we can. The purpose of this book is to show you how to do just that.

CHAPTER 2

HIGH-ENERGY EATING HABITS

What do you eat first thing in the morning? If you're like most Americans, you eat something bready—toast, muffin, bagel, toaster waffle—or a bowl of hot or cold packaged breakfast cereal; maybe a container of fruit-sweetened yogurt. You're a health-conscious person. You know it's a bad idea to skip breakfast.

These options are all quick and tasty, and there is not much mess. You gulp down your coffee or your orange juice, and you're on your way into your busy day.

But then, about 10:00 A.M., you start to feel lightheaded, shaky. You've *got* to get your hands on some carbohydrates. You go to the coffee shop or vending machine to get some calories into your body. You feel better for a little while, but by lunchtime, you're weak, shaky, and ravenous again. After your low-fat salad and breadsticks at lunch, you go through the same energetic ups and downs until dinner—at which time you gorge yourself on pasta. In front of the TV, you continue to nibble well into the evening. You're finally feeling satiated.

Before bed, you get on the scale and see that you've gained another two pounds. Your sleep is fitful and you wake feeling drained the next morning.

What's wrong with this picture? This chapter will fill you in on the mistakes many people make when choosing the foods they eat—mistakes that put them on an energy roller coaster rather than maintaining steady energy throughout the day. You will learn how to design a diet that gently boosts your morning energy levels and maintains them throughout the day.

If you aren't eating right, supplements to boost your energy won't help much. With this in mind, let's talk about high-energy eating habits.

The First Rule of High-Energy Eating: Balancing Protein, Fat, and Carbohydrate

The most important aspect of the high-energy diet is keeping blood sugar levels steady. When you eat sugar and other fast-burning carbohydrates (potatoes, bananas, melon) without protein, your body rapidly breaks those carbohydrates down into glucose, which then goes into your bloodstream. Your pancreas pumps out insulin, which shuttles those blood sugars into the cells to be burned as fuel in mitochondria, or into storage depots in liver and fat cells. You experience a brief burst of energy.

The more intense and rapid the upward surge in blood sugar, the more intense and rapid the corresponding insulin surge. Sugars are depleted from your bloodstream quickly, and you can end up hypoglycemic; in this condition, low blood sugar causes you to feel dizzy, lightheaded, fatigued, or clumsy.

Eating nothing but carbohydrates—especially, simple carbohydrates made from white flour and sugar—is a recipe for energy drain. Adding protein and fiber to the mix will help prevent these ups and downs by slowing the absorption of carbohydrates and their elevating effects on blood sugar.

In the morning, you've been fasting for several hours, and blood sugar levels are low, but your body has settled into a metabolic state that encourages the burning of fats for energy. Once you introduce carbohydrates, you're set up for a day of blood sugar peaks and valleys.

For optimal energy, think *high protein* in the

morning, and increase the proportion of calories from carbohydrate as you move through the day. Try an omelet or scramble made with a small amount of olive oil or butter, three egg whites and one or two yolks, vegetables (mushrooms, spinach, broccoli, whatever you like), and meat if you like (lean turkey, ham, or turkey sausage or bacon, for example). Accompany your main dish with a slice of whole-grain toast or a whole-grain tortilla. Or you can try:

- A cup of plain yogurt with fruit and granola or muesli mixed in; try adding a scoop of protein powder.

- A breakfast burrito on whole-grain tortilla, made with scrambled tofu and egg, herbs, salsa, a little grated cheddar, and raw baby spinach leaves.

- A cup of oatmeal with yogurt and fruit; protein powder will work here too.

- A shake made with egg or whey protein or soft tofu, fruit, and plain yogurt; add some spirulina or other greens powder if you don't mind the color or slightly grassy taste—concentrated greens are very energizing!

Burst free of the conventional American pancakes-toast-eggs-bacon-cereal-for-breakfast paradigm. Try leftovers from the previous night's dinner, or a turkey or tofu burger with melted organic cheese on a slice of whole-grain toast with tomato and lettuce.

> Instead of a double espresso, try a double shot of energy-rich wheat grass juice—available at most juice bars.

Snacking can help maintain energy throughout the day. Avoid high-carbohydrate pastries, candy, and chips. Opt for a combination of a fruit or vegetable with some protein and fat:

- Yogurt or cottage cheese with fruit (add ground flax seeds for fiber).
- Protein smoothie (careful—many sold in juice bars contain a lot of sugar).
- Apple slices or celery sticks with cheese or nut butter.
- Miso soup (usually contains soybean paste, tofu, and scallions).

If this combining of foods seems too complicated, it's best to stick with protein: a hard-boiled egg, a few slices of leftover chicken, turkey, or beef, cheese or baked tofu, or a handful of nuts or seeds, for example. Commercially available high-protein nutrition bars generally contain artificial ingredients and flavorings, but they're a better choice than an 800-calorie white-flour, sugar- glazed muffin.

At lunch and dinner time, keep trying to balance carbs, protein, and fat—intuitively, without making it into a complex mathematical equation. Have a serving of protein (beef, poultry, tofu, beans/ rice, fish) no larger than a deck of cards, some vegetables, and a couple of tablespoons of healthy fat (in an olive oil vinaigrette, for example) or some nuts.

Don't eat too much at one sitting; your body diverts much of its energy to digestion—and away from brain and muscle—after a big meal.

The Second Rule: Curb Your Refined Carbohydrate Consumption

The human body is wired to desire the tastes and textures of highly refined carbohydrates. Our genes developed a taste for sweet food thousands of years ago; food was scarce, and we needed to pack on pounds when food was abundant. It's an uphill battle to turn down refined carbs in favor of less palatable, less calorically dense food, but it's a battle worth fighting. A diet rich in refined carbohydrates—sweets, white bread, sodas—is now believed to do far more than drain energy: it also predisposes us to obesity, diabetes, and heart disease.

Use whole-grain products instead of white flour, and try cooked whole grains—brown rice, quinoa, and barley, for example. Avoid sodas and sweetened coffee drinks, which can pack up to 10 teaspoons of sugar per serving! Instead, try herbal teas, sparkling waters, or organic juices (recent research shows that pomegranate, blueberry, and purple grape juices are especially nourishing) when you want something more flavorful than water. Overindulging in alcoholic beverages can drain your energy, but one glass of wine or beer a day should be fine for most people.

Choose one or two days a week to indulge in a sweet treat instead of making sugar a dietary staple.

The Third Rule: Eat Your Colors

The more naturally colorful the foods you eat, the more packed they are with nutrients that will promote energy and clarity. When you fill your plate, try to combine as many colors as you can: reds, oranges, greens, yellows, purples, browns. For example, try a filet of deep, pink wild-caught salmon with a bunch of deep green broccoli and bright yellow corn on the cob. Or a plate of spinach pasta with ruby-red peppers and tomatoes sautéed in olive oil with garlic and onions; or brown rice, chicken, and a big vegetable salad. Indulge your inner artist!

Antioxidant phytochemicals, vitamins, and minerals are the cogs, wheels, and sparks that make cellular metabolism go. Eating a diet that gets its varied hues from nature—not the white-flour, bland, artificially colored diets on which so many

Americans subsist—guarantees that your body will have its basic nutritional and metabolic needs met.

The Fourth Rule:
Stop Eating Early in the Evening

Do you almost always skip breakfast—either because you are not hungry, or because you feel guilty about having eaten too much the night before? Do you eat more after dinner than you do during dinner, or more than half your day's food intake during and following dinner? Do you get up from a deep sleep in the middle of the night to have something to eat? And do you munch away during evening hours on high-carbohydrate sugars and starches, feeling shame and anxiety about the whole business?

According to recent psychiatric research, this pattern—when persisting for two or more months—is indicative of *night-eating syndrome* (NES). This constellation of symptoms is common in obese people (one study estimates that over one-quarter of people who are 100 pounds or more overweight have NES), and is believed to be related to difficulty coping with stress and tension. Anxiety, agitation, and insomnia are commonly experienced along with other aspects of this so-called syndrome. Unlike binge eating, which is done in short episodes, night-eating syndrome is a constant grazing throughout the night.

Some research suggests that NES is linked with overproduction of cortisol, which causes carbohydrate cravings, particularly in the evening. Refined carbohydrates can alter neurotransmitter systems in a mood-boosting direction almost as deftly as a drug can, and a person whose stresses start to overwhelm them in the evening hours can feel better after eating a high-carb snack. In other words, night eating may

Cortisol
A hormome produced by the adrenal glands; commonly called the stress hormone.

be a way of "self-medicating," according to the experts at Anorexia Nervosa and Related Eating Disorders, Inc.

Even those who don't have the complete set of NES symptoms may tend to eat most of their calories at dinner and afterward. This can sap your energy, as it makes for less restful sleep—your body is hard at work digesting all that food during the hours it needs all possible energy to regenerate and renew—and often leads to weight gain.

Spread your calories out over the day. Stop eating once the dinner dishes are cleared. Going to bed a little hungry is probably best. Then, in the morning, you'll have an appetite for a hearty breakfast.

The Fifth Rule:
Eat Raw Food as Often as Possible

Raw food is living food. It contains enzymes and nutrients that become depleted with cooking. Any food subjected to temperatures above 110°F will lose its enzyme activity and some of its nutritional value. Enzymes in food enhance energy by doing some of the work of breaking down food in your gut. Your body conserves some of the energy required for digestion and assimilation.

Some health educators advise the consumption of a completely raw diet—no cooked food whatsoever. The mainstay of such a diet is fruit and vegetables, with specially prepared sprouted grains, seeds, and nuts. It is a spartan regimen, but people who can pull it off tend to have more energy than they know what to do with—at least, for a few weeks. Raw food diets are cleansing and, because they are low in calories, don't put a lot of stress on the body. You're likely to settle into a metabolic state that relies on burning mostly fat.

Eating only raw food isn't a regimen we recommend long term, because it's so extreme. Depletion and weakness are common after longer periods on this diet. Simply adding some raw food to each meal will make a difference in your energy level. Spinach leaves, apple, carrot, celery, fresh berries, tomato slices, cucumber, onion, alfalfa or other sprouts . . . the choices are endless! Of course, raw meat is a terrible idea, although raw fish—at a sushi bar, or sushi-grade bought at your market—is highly nutritious and energizing.

Eat about 40 to 50 percent raw food in the summer, and 25 percent in the winter (in some areas, you may not be able to find much fresh produce during the winter). Raw food's enzyme content is highest soon after harvesting. The fresher your produce, the more energizing it will be to your body.

The Sixth Rule: TLC for Your Digestive Tract

Your digestive tract is the first link in the chain of events that transforms food and nutrients into energy. The standard American diet (SAD) is very tough on the gastrointestinal system. It's low in fiber and water, which tends to result in constipation—a condition that can make you tired, particularly if it's chronic. The SAD is high in refined sugars, which breed unfriendly yeasts that can cause digestive difficulties.

Stomach acids have gotten a lot of bad press because of the epidemic of gastroesophageal reflux disease (GERD)—a fancy name for chronic heartburn. Food mixed with stomach acid is "burped" back up past the entrance to the stomach, burning the lining of the esophagus. Antacids or acid-inhibiting drugs are commonly used to counter this problem—however, according to some experts, using them can do more harm than good.

There is evidence that the problem in many people who have chronic heartburn is not too much stomach acid, but too *little*. Acid starts the process of breaking food down in the stomach, and the contents of the stomach have to reach the proper pH to open the sphincter into the small intestines—a fail-safe method that prevents food from passing into that long, winding tube before it's been broken down adequately. If there's too little acid, and the food sits there too long, some of it may start to back up.

Diets composed mostly of cooked food require the pancreas—which makes digestive enzymes in addition to insulin—to crank out extra enzymes to ensure that food is broken down all the way, into the form in which nutrients can be absorbed into the bloodstream and distributed to tissues. And the SAD tends to be low in *fructooligosaccharides* (FOS), which are the preferred food of the friendly probiotic bacteria that live in our GI tracts and aid in proper digestion. FOS are found in fruit, vegetables, and whole grains.

Aid your digestive tract in liberating energy from the food you eat, by:

- Taking small bites and chewing the food thoroughly, until it is liquefied in your mouth.

- Avoiding ice-cold drinks with food; this can slow down digestion.

- Eating raw food with every meal and snack, if possible.

- Eating foods fermented with friendly probiotics—best known for their role in transforming milk into yogurt, but also used, for example, to make miso out of soy and sauerkraut out of cabbage. Or, supplement your daily diet with a living probiotic in capsule form.

- Trying natural ways to control GERD, heartburn, or indigestion: chew or swallowing an enzyme tablet, containing protease, lipase, cellulase, and other digestive enzymes, with your meals; before eating, drink down a cup of room-temperature water mixed with two tablespoons of apple cider vinegar.

- Dealing with constipation by increasing fiber and fluid intake. Psyllium and ground flaxseed should work, but the best way to improve "regularity" is to drastically increase the amount of vegetables you eat—and exercise daily!

- Breaking the pattern of caffeine dependency. A cup of coffee in the morning is okay, but gulping down triple cappuccinos two or three times a day just to stay awake at your desk isn't. Tapped-out adrenals could result if you continue to rely on caffeine for energy.

- Adding "green foods" (chlorella, spirulina, blue-green algae, wheat- or barley grass juice) to your diet to help relieve constipation, improve liver function, and supply plentiful energy-boosting nutrients.

Concluding Thoughts on an Energy-Boosting Diet

Food *is* energy. From the bottom of the food chain (algae) to the top (you and me), the process of eating and being eaten is all about the storage and transfer of energy from one being to another.

It's nice when food tastes good, but its primary role is to fuel your body's energy-making machinery. Many of us are fortunate enough to have the best of both worlds available to us: we can eat food that's nourishing, energizing—*and* delicious!

CHAPTER 3

CELL ENERGY:
COENZYME Q_{10}

If one nutrient had been shown to be useful for the prevention or treatment of heart failure, high blood pressure, cancer, AIDS, Parkinson's disease, Huntington's disease, mitochondrial diseases, and chronic fatigue . . . well, you'd have heard about it by now. Right?

Maybe not. There is just such a nutrient: coenzyme Q_{10}, also known as *ubiquinone* because of its ubiquitous presence in living cells. Strong research evidence supports its use as a therapy for some of the most challenging illnesses of modern times. And yet, if you were to ask the average doctor whether she recommends its use to her patients, she'd likely say, "Coenzyme *what?*"

Coenzyme Q_{10}—CoQ_{10} for short—is a substance found in nature. It is in many of the foods we eat, although in small concentrations. (To take in the minimum recommended 30-milligram dose of CoQ_{10} from food, you'd have to eat a pound of sardines, two pounds of beef, or two and a half pounds of peanuts!) It is found most abundantly in the tissues of the heart, kidney, brain, muscle, and liver.

In order to cover the costs of creating and spreading the word to doctors about any new treatment, drug companies—physicians' main source of information about new treatments—have to be able to patent new products. As a natural substance, CoQ_{10} cannot be patented. This is why your doctor has most likely not heard about it, or doesn't know enough about it to recommend it to you.

This tide may be turning, however—at least where CoQ_{10} is concerned—because of the effects of popular cholesterol-lowering drugs on levels of this nutrient in the body. Doctors are well-versed in pharmaceutical cholesterol-lowering therapies—at least 12 million Americans take them, and current recommendations are pushing for nearly triple that number to start. But these therapies may pose great risks because of their effects on the body's ability to make adequate coenzyme Q_{10}. If your doctor *has* heard of CoQ_{10}, it is most likely in the context of the risks of statin drugs.

Statin Drugs
Pharmaceuticals that inhibit the action of an enzyme needed to make cholesterol.

CoQ_{10} and Statin Drug Side Effects

Heart muscle cells contain very high concentrations of coenzyme Q_{10}, and for good reason: beating 100,000 times a day for a lifetime requires some high-end metabolic machinery, and heart cells need plentiful CoQ_{10} to run that machinery. Depletions of CoQ_{10} in the heart muscle reduce its pumping strength.

There is a natural age-related decline in CoQ_{10} levels in the heart and elsewhere—a decline that is believed to begin in our forties and that, by age ninety, brings levels of CoQ_{10} in the mitochondria down to only 5 percent of what they were in our youth. Risk of heart failure rises with aging, and one pivotal factor may be CoQ_{10} depletion.

The effects of popular *HMG co-A reductase (HMG Co-A) inhibitor* drugs (also known as statins) on CoQ_{10} levels in the body, and the effects of that drug-induced CoQ_{10} lack on the health of the heart, are a good illustration of the importance of this underappreciated nutrient.

Statins inhibit the action of an enzyme necessary for the formation of cholesterol—an enzyme that also happens to be required for the synthesis of coenzyme Q_{10}. Taking these drugs will lower body levels of this nutrient, and it looks like this has potentially serious consequences.

Statins are very effective at lowering cholesterol, but for years, research hasn't shown that they are as protective against heart disease as they were expected to be—and that they could cause some disconcerting side effects:

- They seemed to protect middle-aged users with high cholesterol, but not elderly people, against heart disease.

- Statins can cause a rare and potentially fatal side effect called rhabdomyolysis; in this condition, muscle tissue breaks down and the resulting release of protein into the bloodstream overloads the kidneys.

- Mild muscle pain and weakness are common side effects with statin therapy. One study found that statin users who complained of muscle pain had *iatrogenic* (caused by medical care) mitochondrial myopathy, which went away when the drugs were stopped.

- Increased risk of heart failure and impairment of the heart's pumping function has been found in some research on statins. It looks as though statins help keep the blood vessels that feed the heart muscle clear—but can diminish the heart's pumping strength.

- A large-scale clinical trial found a 25 percent increase in cancer incidence in patients age seventy and older who were using statins, compared with a matched placebo group. This was not a complete surprise; statins had previously been reported to cause cancer in animals.

As you continue to read through this chapter, you will see that every one of these side effects from statin drugs could well be due—at least, in part—to their effects on coenzyme Q_{10} production. Some drug companies are, at this writing, beginning to look into adding CoQ_{10} to their statin formulations.

CoQ_{10}: History and Present-Day Perspectives

Coenzyme Q_{10} was discovered in 1957. Its role in cellular energy production was fully described four years later by the University of Edinburgh's Peter Mitchell, Ph.D.—an achievement that won Dr. Mitchell a Nobel prize for chemistry. Further research demonstrated that coenzyme Q_{10} does double duty, acting not only as a cog in the wheel of cellular energy production, but also as a powerful antioxidant. It is this combination of roles that makes CoQ_{10} an amazing therapeutic agent for a wide range of conditions.

Two roles of CoQ_{10} have been established. First, it is used by cells to produce energy in the mitochondria. It transfers energy, in the form of electrons, from complexes I and II of the mitochondrial respiratory chain to complex III.

Its secondary role in the body is as an antioxidant. It can be incorporated into cholesterol molecules, helping to prevent them from becoming oxidized by free radicals and thus contributing to increased risk of heart disease. (Trustworthy experts maintain that the overall level of cholesterol is a less important contributor to heart disease than whether that cholesterol is oxidized.) CoQ_{10} also protects the delicate membranes that surround each cell against free radical attack.

This is a handy double-duty for a nutrient to play—it's in the thick of energy production, which produces excess free radicals; and it helps to "mop up" those free radicals with its antioxidant power.

Mental cloudiness, gingivitis, weakness, fatigue, and lactic acidosis (where lactic acid accumulates because cells are relying on glycolysis) are seen in severe CoQ$_{10}$ deficiency. Low levels of CoQ$_{10}$ are seen in people with cardiovascular disease, some cancers, hypertension (high blood pressure), periodontal disease, AIDS, Parkinson's disease, diabetes, and congestive heart failure (CHF). Aging and CoQ$_{10}$ levels are linked.

As soon as the research community sees common ground between lack of a nutrient and disease, studies begin to seek whether there might be some causal connection, and whether supplementing with that nutrient might help with disease prevention or control. With CoQ$_{10}$, most research explored the link between CoQ$_{10}$ deficiency and heart failure, with some additional research into the use of this nutrient as a complementary therapy for cancer, gingivitis/periodontal disease, and loss of energy and strength in aging people. Eight international symposia have been held on the use of CoQ$_{10}$ for heart failure and other illnesses; more than three hundred studies presented there reinforced the promise of this energy-boosting nutrient.

CoQ$_{10}$ for Heart Failure

Heart failure is an extreme form of energy deficiency at the cellular level. The heart muscle becomes damaged by heart attack or by viral or bacterial infection. Sometimes, the reason for the damage to the heart is unknown—*idiopathic*, in medical-speak. Whatever the cause, the result is the same: a weakened, enlarged heart muscle that can't efficiently pump blood out to the rest of the body. The heart's shape gradually changes in an effort to pump more blood, which in the end decreases its efficiency further. Oxidative stress increases dramatically in a failing heart, and levels of coenzyme Q$_{10}$ fall.

Oxidation
The formation of free radicals, which damage cells.

It is believed by CoQ_{10} researchers that in some cases of heart failure, deficiency of coenzyme Q_{10} is the primary cause of the problem. Since the late 1990s, studies have demonstrated that coenzyme Q_{10} supplementation can be highly beneficial to heart failure patients. In some cases, it has completely reversed the disease; in others, it has helped patients reduce the number of drugs they needed.

According to coenzyme Q_{10} researcher Peter Langsjöen, M.D., " . . . [D]eficiency of CoQ_{10} appears to be a major treatable factor in the otherwise inexorable progression of heart disease . . . The clinical experience with CoQ_{10} in heart failure is nothing short of dramatic, and it is reasonable to believe that the entire field of medicine should be re-evaluated in light of this growing knowledge."

Most of the research into CoQ_{10} for heart failure has been done in Japan, with some from the United States, Germany, Italy, and Sweden. The studies uniformly show that CoQ_{10} improves *ejection fraction,* the amount of blood the heart pumps out with each beat; yields a gradual, sustained improvement in the heartbeat's regularity; and reduces fatigue, shortness of breath, heart palpitations, and chest pains. These kinds of improvements have generally been observed in a high percentage of patients who took CoQ_{10}, while placebo patients stayed the same or got worse.

Most remarkable in studies of CoQ_{10} therapy for heart failure was the impact on patients' quality of life. Heart failure is no picnic, and improvements are hard-won. Patients may require multiple drugs that cause major side effects. CoQ_{10} therapy has been documented to reduce the need for drugs in heart failure patients, enhance their energy, and reduce fatigue.

Strong evidence suggests that people who take statin drugs can decrease their risk of heart failure by taking CoQ_{10} daily.

Can CoQ$_{10}$ Prevent Heart Disease?

Atherosclerosis, a process in which damaged blood vessels around the heart develop fatty "caps" that can then partially or completely cut off blood flow to the heart muscle—an event known as a heart attack—is what scientists call a *multifactorial* disease. Several risk factors exist, and the more of these risk factors you have, the more likely you are to end up suffering a heart attack. The combination that puts you most at risk: high blood pressure and high insulin and blood sugar levels (all of which can damage the walls of blood vessels) and elevated "bad" LDL cholesterol counts with low HDL.

Handling multiple risk factors can require a rather extensive pharmaceutical arsenal, including statins for cholesterol, diuretics or other drugs for hypertension, glucose-lowering drugs for high glucose and insulin level, and possibly additional drugs to help thin the blood. Many people end up on regimens involving daily doses of three or more medicines each day. One of the major side effects of medicines used to prevent heart attacks is fatigue—and lack of CoQ$_{10}$ could well be a major contributing factor to that picture.

An eight-week study performed by researchers in the country Georgia compared two groups of patients who were using statins to prevent atherosclerosis: one group used 60 milligrams of CoQ$_{10}$ daily, and the other only took the drug (simvastatin). The statin-plus-CoQ$_{10}$ group had significant reductions in free radical measurements, an increase in the blood fats that are protective against heart disease, and less "sticky" blood (stickier blood is more likely to clot and block narrowed blood vessels).

A study by Peter Langsjöen and coworkers enrolled 109 patients with hypertension and gave them daily doses of CoQ$_{10}$. After about four and a half months, 51 percent of the patients were able to stop taking between one and three drugs for their hypertension. Langsjöen theorizes that the reduction in blood pressure with CoQ_{10} is likely due to improvements in *diastolic function*—the part of the heartbeat where it expands to bring blood into itself. A stiffening of the heart muscle walls, often seen with aging, interferes with diastolic function, and CoQ_{10} has been found to help reverse this change.

In the end, CoQ_{10} looks like it could help control several of the risk factors for heart attack.

CoQ_{10} and Lack of Energy in Aging People

Remember that aging gradually reduces mitochondrial efficiency. After age thirty or forty, defects in mitochondrial DNA increase, especially in muscle, heart, and brain, where CoQ_{10} is most abundant. This translates to a functional deficiency of this nutrient that appears to be replaceable with supplementation.

CoQ_{10} has been found to enhance the effects of enzymes that are responsible for repairing damaged DNA—a major cause of mitochondrial dysfunction with aging. CoQ_{10} has been found to protect mitochondrial DNA in mice who were given a drug that causes high levels of oxidative stress.

Studies of old and young rodent heart cells found, not surprisingly, that older heart cells contracted less strongly than young heart cells during simulated exercise stress. After six weeks of CoQ_{10} supplementation, the old hearts had *four times* the work capacity of the young hearts! According to researcher Anthony Linnane, "age-related differences in contractile power of heart cells was abolished by CoQ_{10}." Current research shows that diastolic function is markedly improved in elderly people (average age of eighty-four years), with

accompanying improvements in exercise tolerance and quality of life.

CoQ$_{10}$ for Chronic Fatigue

Complaints of devastating fatigue and other mys-
terious symptoms, including vertigo, for six months
or more can lead to a diagnosis of chronic fatigue
syndrome (CFS).

   In a study performed at the University of Iowa's
College of Medicine, researchers gathered 155
subjects who had unexplained chronic fatigue for
months or years. They were tracked for six months
to two years as they tried nutritional and medical
treatments and lifestyle changes to try to regain
their health. The treatments that the patients felt
worked best to relieve their fatigue were coenzyme Q$_{10}$ (69 percent of thirteen subjects who
tried it experienced a lift in their energy levels); the
hormone DHEA; and the herb ginseng, which is
covered in depth later in this book. Multivitamins,
vigorous exercise, and yoga also proved helpful in
this study.

CoQ$_{10}$ and Cancer

Once a cell becomes cancerous,
its energy production changes—it
relies primarily on glycolysis. This
makes it highly energy inefficient,
a cellular energy hog. In the disease's advanced stages, tumors use
up most of the energy in the body,
leading to fat loss and muscle
wasting known as *cachexia*.

Cachexia
*General weight
loss and muscle
wasting character-
istic of certain
diseases.*

   Some research suggests that cachexia can be
counteracted by CoQ$_{10}$ supplementation. Other
studies have found that CoQ$_{10}$ encourages cancer
cell death and potently inhibits cancer growth.

   In his article on CoQ$_{10}$, Nutrition Reporter Jack
Challem describes the phenomenal results of a
study by Karl Folkers, one of the original CoQ$_{10}$

researchers: "Folkers described 10 cancer patients given CoQ_{10} for heart failure. One of the patients, a 48-year-old man diagnosed in 1977 with inoperable lung cancer, has not had any signs of either cancer or heart failure symptoms while taking CoQ_{10} for 17 years."

Many studies involving CoQ_{10} and cancer incorporate antioxidants, essential fatty acids, and other supplements. One such study by Knud Lockwood, M.D., a Danish oncologist, found that thirty-two women with aggressive breast cancer all survived the disease through the 24 months of the study—and the therapy dramatically improved their well-being. (Statistically, six deaths would be expected within that time frame.) Dr. Lockwood was amazed to see spontaneous, complete regression of 1.5 to 2.0 centimeter breast tumors—which he had never seen with conventional therapies—in patients who took CoQ_{10} and other nutrients.

In 2005, the University of Miami's Miller School of Medicine performed studies in their laboratory that showed CoQ_{10} to be a potent inhibitor of breast and prostate cancer cell growth. According to lead researcher Niven Nardin, M.D., the nutrient appeared to "restore [the] cancer cell's ability to kill itself while not impacting normal cells." In the future, cancer treatment could include topical, injected, or swallowed coenzyme Q_{10}.

CoQ_{10} Wrap-Up

This nutrient has other potential applications—too many to fit into this chapter in detail. It shows promise as a treatment for migraine, Parkinson's disease, Huntington's chorea, and AIDS. Diabetics may benefit from its use, too. Periodontal disease is characterized by low CoQ_{10} levels, and restoring optimum levels of this nutrient is one of the most effective natural cures for this problem.

No significant side effects have ever been reported with CoQ_{10}, even with high doses. It has been found to reduce the effectiveness of the anti-coagulant drug warfarin (Coumadin); if you are on this drug, consult your doctor before trying CoQ_{10}. CoQ_{10} may reduce your needs for heart medications, so have your healthcare provider monitor your progress as you use this nutrient.

How to Use Coenzyme Q10

If you are in good health, try 30 to 100 milligrams per day of CoQ_{10}. Take it with a fat-containing food, such as buttered (whole-grain) bread, eggs, fatty fish, or nut butter to improve its absorption.

If you have cardiac risk factors or periodontal disease, or use statin drugs, try 100 milligrams per day. If you have cancer, heart failure, heart disease, or cardiomyopathy (enlarged heart), talk with your healthcare provider about using doses anywhere from 30 to 400 or more milligrams per day.

CHAPTER 4

SAFE ENERGY: ALPHA-LIPOIC ACID

Picture two cages housing lab rats. In one cage are old rats, aged between twenty-four and twenty-eight months; in the next cage, young rats, newbies only two to four weeks old.

The old rats are tired and feeble, with dull coats and bald spots. They creep to their chow bowls, sip a little water, and do a bit of digging and scratching, but the thrill is gone. They perform poorly when white-coated humans test their memory power. Overall, they have a third of the energy and vigor of their younger counterparts—who frolic and canoodle in the adjacent cage just as the old rats did in their glory days.

Then, the white-coated humans start to add one secret ingredient to the old rats' chow, and another to their water. A few days go by, then a few weeks, and some remarkable changes begin to happen. The old rats' physical activity begins to match that of rats less than half their age. Their performance on tests of memory improve. This magical ingredient appears to actually *reverse* the rats' aging. Deeper analysis reveals that the aged rats' mitochondria are working like those of much younger rodents.

I'm describing here a study by Bruce Ames, Ph.D., who stated after the study's publication that "with the two supplements . . . these old rats got up and did the Macarena . . . the brain looks better, they are full of energy—everything we looked at looks like a young animal." The age-reversing effects of these supplements was equivalent to turning the clock of a seventy-five- or eighty-five-year-old human back to middle age.

The two supplements used by Dr. Ames, a professor of molecular and cell biology at the University of California, Berkeley, and his research colleagues were alpha-lipoic acid (ALA) and acetyl-L-carnitine (ALC).

Mitochondrial Deterioration as the "Weak Link in Aging"

According to Dr. Ames, one of the first scientists to talk about the role of free radicals in disease and the potential protective role of antioxidants, mitochondria are the "weak link in aging."

Accumulated free radicals in mitochondria end up gumming up the works of cellular metabolism. With the combination therapy of ALA and ALC, Ames believed he could quench the overflow of damaging free radicals (with ALA) while enhancing the activity of an enzyme—*carnitine acetyl-transferase*—that is an important tool for energy production in the mitochondria (with ALC). In his many studies on this supplement combination, he obtained results beyond his expectations.

Carnitine will be addressed in detail in Chapter 5 . For now, let's turn our attention to the other half of Dr. Ames's anti-aging cocktail: alpha-lipoic acid.

Alpha-Lipoic Acid 101

First discovered in 1951, alpha-lipoic acid was revealed to be a powerful antioxidant in the late 1980s. Specifically, it was found to neutralize *peroxynitrite* radicals, which are implicated in heart and lung disease, neurological disorders, and chronic inflammation.

ALA is made in the mitochondria, where it serves multiple functions in the Krebs cycle. In the liver, it promotes the activity of detoxification enzymes that help to rid the body of toxins, including natural byproducts of metabolism. Like Coenzyme Q_{10},

ALA can be an effective treatment for mitochondrial myopathies.

Alpha-lipoic acid is a uniquely versatile antioxidant; it works in both the fatty and watery parts of
cells. (Most antioxidants are either water soluble,
like vitamin C, or fat soluble, like vitamin E.) Nor-
mally, available alpha-lipoic acid in the cells is used
in the Krebs cycle; supplemental ALA avails your
body of extra amounts that go toward antioxidant
activity.

When an antioxidant like vitamin C or vitamin
E quenches a free radical, it becomes oxidized
itself—in other words, a "spent" antioxidant becomes a free radical. This helps to explain why clinical studies of high doses of single antioxidants
often have contradictory results: antioxidants need
to work cooperatively, trading electrons and regen-
erating one another, to avoid a situation where
oxidative burden ends up increasing. This doesn't
happen with ALA, which generously passes out
electrons to rejuvenate those spent antioxidants.
In this way, ALA's antioxidant action is exponential
in nature.

ALA increases levels of another antioxidant, *glutathione*, in
the cells. Glutathione is made in
the body from the amino acid
cysteine. ALA helps move more
cysteine into the cells, inducing
increased production of glutathione there. Oxidized glutathione can be rejuvenated by ALA.

Glutathione

*An antioxidant
that is instrumental in
protecting the liver
and other body
tissues from
oxidation.*

ALA Is Easily Absorbed and Nontoxic

ALA is very well absorbed in the gut, and is rapidly converted in tissues to usable and potent forms.
It is nontoxic.

Plants and animals both contain alpha-lipoic
acid, but the only appreciable dietary source is red
meat. Since red meat isn't something we want to

eat a whole lot of, supplements are the best way to add extra ALA to your diet.

ALA for Diabetic Complications

Diabetes is, at its root, a problem of energy production. Fatigue is often one of the first signs of its onset.

ALA has been used as a drug in Germany since the late 1980s to treat *peripheral neuropathy*, a common consequence of diabetes. In peripheral neuropathy, chronically high circulating levels of sugar in the blood cause damage to nerves in the legs and feet.

Both type 1 and type 2 diabetes can cause neuropathies. In type 1 diabetes, which usually develops in young children, the hormone insulin isn't made in the pancreas in amounts adequate to usher glucose out of the bloodstream and into the cells. Insulin injections are necessary for life.

In type 2 diabetes, a combination of obesity and genetic predisposition cause body cells to stop hearing the "knock-knock" of insulin as it tries to move glucose in. This condition, called *insulin resistance*, may exist for some time before full-blown diabetes sets in. Blood glucose levels rise, but cells are starved for fuel: type 2 diabetes has been called "starvation in the midst of plenty."

If caught early, type 2 diabetes can be reversed with weight loss, healthful diet, and exercise (which moves glucose into cells without the help of insulin). But, when type 2 diabetes progresses unaddressed, the pancreas keeps trying to pump out more insulin to overcome cells' resistance. Glucose and insulin levels rise to dangerous heights, damaging blood vessels and nerves as they increase oxidation and glycation in the tissues. Glucose-lowering drugs—and, potentially, insulin injections, once the pancreas has exhausted itself—may become nec-

Glycation
The process in which sugars are bound to proteins.

essary. All in all, a bad scene, and most certainly an energy-draining one.

If today's diabetes problem is any indication, and if ALA is as good a diabetes fighter as the research shows it to be, this supplement is poised to become a highly important alternative therapy.

The Diabetes Epidemic: Could ALA Help?

Statistics from 2002 found that 18.3 million Americans had been diagnosed with type 2 diabetes. According to the World Health Organization, more than 150 million are believed to be affected worldwide. According to the website www.wrongdiag nosis.com, some 5 million people who have the disease don't know it. It's commonly misdiagnosed or undiagnosed.

Also widely acknowledged is a condition known variously as "the metabolic syndrome" or Syndrome X—the constellation of risk factors that leads to diabetes:

- Obesity, particularly in and around the abdominal area.

- Imbalanced blood fats, with high triglycerides and low "good" HDL cholesterol.

- Insulin resistance, where cells become less sensitive to insulin and blood glucose doesn't readily pass into cells.

- "Thickened" blood, with high measurements of clotting factors.

- Hypertension (130/85 mm Hg or higher).

- Elevated inflammation in the body, measured by the C-reactive protein test.

Statistics from the American Heart Association state that 20 to 25 percent of Americans are believed to have the metabolic syndrome. Fatigue may be the red flag that lets the potential diabetic know that it is time to make drastic changes before it's too late.

A weight-reduction diet that is dense with anti-oxidant nutrients and that centers on whole food with few to no refined carbohydrates or sugar will also reduce blood pressure and insulin resistance. This diet, along with nutritional supplements that reduce blood clotting (most notably, vitamin E and fish oil), can help head off many of the problems characteristic of Syndrome X before they get severe. Daily aerobic exercise is just as important as changing your diet.

ALA has been found to speed the movement of glucose from the bloodstream into cells by improving the function of insulin. It has been shown in several studies to reduce insulin resistance —at least in part by increasing the permeability of cell membranes; this permeability is reduced by high blood sugar.

Permeability
A measurement of how easily a substance can pass through a barrier.

A study of obese, diabetic mice found that ALA increased glucose uptake from 40 percent to 300 percent. In another study, researchers demonstrated that diabetics' blood lactic acid and pyruvate levels dropped with ALA supplementation.

Paraesthesiae
Burning, tickling, or other uncomfortable sensations.

Studies show that 600 milligrams of ALA per day can reduce pain, burning, paraesthesiae, and numbness in the legs and feet of people with type 2 diabetes. ALA improves blood circulation to nerves, which are often affected by neuropathy, and it also promotes healthy dilation of blood vessels.

ALA's Anti-Aging Appeal

As you learned earlier in this chapter, studies suggest that ALA may well be in the water at the fabled fountain of youth. Here's a sampling of some of the fascinating research being done on this nutrient:

- Researchers in India found that "[m]itochondria from aged tissue use oxygen inefficiently, impairing ATP synthesis and resulting in increased oxidant production," and that ALA-supplemented rats had significant increases in levels of Krebs cycle enzymes and antioxidants (C, E, and glutathione) at the cellular level.

- A study published in the journal *Proceedings of the National Academy of Sciences* in 2002 showed that memory loss in old rats was associated with mitochondrial decay and DNA oxidation in the brain—and that supplementing the rats with the "magical" ALA/ALC cocktail, or either nutrient separately, could partially reverse these changes.

- Another rat study, this one from the Linus Pauling Institute in Corvallis, Oregon, measured oxidative stress, free radical production, antioxidant status, and oxidative DNA damage in the hearts of young rats twenty-eight-months old and two-months old. Old rats had almost three times the free radical production and a twofold decline in vitamin C levels compared with the young rats. The older rats had much more free radical–caused DNA damage in their heart cells. After supplementing some of the rats' food with ALA, it was found that the hearts of old rats on ALA had a markedly lower rate of free radical production—a rate that matched that of unsupplemented young rats. Vitamin C levels rose and oxidative DNA damage was reduced in the old rats on ALA.

ALA Spells . . . Energy?

Maybe not, but this nutrient has a huge amount of research push behind it. No study has shown it to be dangerous, even in high doses—although diabetics should be carefully monitored while using ALA, because their needs for medication or insulin are likely to be reduced. They could end up with *low* blood sugar before adjusting their meds!

If you are diabetic or prediabetic, take 200 milligrams two to three times daily. If you are suffering from neuropathy, the three-times-daily dosing is appropriate. For general protection against free radical damage in healthy people, and to preserve brain and heart function with aging, 100 milligrams twice a day should be adequate.

CHAPTER 5

SLOW ENERGY: CARNITINE AND ACETYL-L-CARNITINE

After finding that a combination of alpha-lipoic acid and acetyl-L-carnitine could rouse old, tired rats from torpor and inspire them to do trendy dances, Dr. Ames gushed that "the animals seem to have much more vigor and are much more active than animals not on this diet, signaling massive improvement to these animals' health and well-being."

Dr. Ames and a colleague, Bruce Hagen, created a patented combination of the two nutrients and founded a company called Juvenon through which to sell it. Human trials that seek to replicate those done with animals are underway at this writing.

Maybe someday soon, it will cease to be unusual to spot seventy-five- and eighty-year-olds engaging in physically demanding pastimes once reserved for younger, more energetic people!

The Role of Carnitine in Metabolism

Although carnitine is made in the body, the need for this nutrient can outstrip production—particularly in people who are on dialysis, are diabetic, have cirrhosis of the liver, or who use certain medications (the anticonvulsant valproic acid; drugs used for AIDS treatment, including zidovudine, also called AZT, didanosine, zalcitabine, and stavudine; and the chemotherapy drugs ifosfamide and cisplatin), or who have problems absorbing adequate nutrients from the food they eat. Because need can exceed the body's capacity to produce it, carnitine is referred to as a *conditionally essential* nutrient.

Kidney dialysis patients are often carnitine deficient, leading to anemia, muscle weakness, and fatigue; the FDA has approved the use of L-carnitine for these patients. Diabetics with complications such as neuropathy have higher likelihood of carnitine deficiency.

Carnitine needs rise during stressful periods and during pregnancy and breastfeeding. This nutrient is found most abundantly in dairy and red meat; people who avoid these foods may need a little extra in supplemental form.

Derived from the amino acids lysine and methionine, and made with the help of vitamins C and B_6, niacin, and iron, carnitine is made primarily in the liver and kidneys. It is transported from there to other parts of the body. The highest body concentration of carnitine is in the skeletal muscles (like those in the arms, legs, and abdomen) and the heart muscle—tissues that prefer to use fat as their primary fuel.

Fat is, by far, the densest source of energy available to cells. One molecule of glucose yields 42 ATP in the Krebs cycle and oxygen transport chain, but a single 18-carbon fatty acid molecule releases 147 ATP as it goes through these processes. Fatty acid metabolism does require more oxygen, but in the end, it releases about the same number of ATP per oxygen molecule. To have abundant energy, your cells need to be able to access and "burn" fats as fuel, both at rest and during mild to moderate exercise.

Outside the mitochondria, carnitine made in the liver or kidneys binds to a fatty acid, and then a transporter made from protein moves it across the inner mitochondrial membrane. There, the fatty acid plus carnitine go through beta-oxidation, yielding energy and end products that can be recycled and used again.

Once inside the mitochondria, carnitine also moves excess intermediates out through the mitochondrial membrane, preventing their accumulation that can gum up the works. Think of carnitine as a metabolic doorman, politely escorting fatty acids in and waste products out of the mitochondria. It also has the fringe benefit of lending support to the benefits of both coenzyme Q_{10} and alpha-lipoic acid—another indication that these three antioxidants work best when they're all used together.

Vitamin C is needed for the production of carnitine. One of the first symptoms of vitamin C deficiency is fatigue, arising as carnitine production slows down and muscles become unable to burn fats efficiently.

Carnitine levels in the tissues decline with age in both humans and animals. This could explain why studies using this nutrient show such dramatic rejuvenative effects with supplementation, at both the whole-body and mitochondrial levels.

The acetyl-L form of carnitine is slightly different from carnitine alone. It has an *acetyl group* attached, and that acetyl group breaks off and can be used as raw material for the neurotransmitter *acetylcholine*. Another form, propionyl-L-carnitine, has also been studied; propionyl-L-carnitine appears slightly better for people with cardiovascular diseases, while the acetyl form appears most effective at promoting better brain function.

Carnitine Helps Prevent Damage from Heart Attacks

When blood flow through a heart vessel is blocked, the tissue downstream of the blockage becomes *ischemic*—deprived of oxygen. This rapidly causes damage that can be permanent. Studies find that pretreating lab rats with L-carnitine reduces heart injury following ischemia.

Giving 4 grams per day of carnitine to humans,

starting just after a heart attack diagnosis, significantly reduced mortality in the year that followed: only 1.2 percent of the carnitine users died in that year, while 12.5 percent of the control subjects died. Heart pains, also called *angina,* were less frequent in carnitine users. Adding 2 grams per day of carnitine to medicines for angina have been found to improve heart failure patients' ability to exercise, and have led to positive changes in electrocardiogram (ECG) measurements of heart function during exercise.

Other studies of humans involving very high-dose intravenous carnitine just following heart attack, with long-term supplementation following, found that this therapy reduced heart enlargement, a common consequence of heart attack. In a preliminary study, patients with diabetes and high blood pressure who took 4 grams of L-carnitine a day had reduced incidence of irregular heartbeat, with reduction in heart function irregularities.

One study found that propionyl-L-carnitine at a dose of 500 milligrams a day significantly increased heart failure patients' exercise tolerance and their ability to take in and use oxygen during exercise.

Sometimes, blood vessel "clogs" arise in areas of the body besides the heart. If in the legs, these clogs—which can cause painful ischemia in the hips, lower legs, or feet—is referred to as *claudication.* In 495 patients with severe claudication, 2 grams per day of propionyl-L-carnitine for 12 months helped them increase the distance they could walk before pain stopped them. Other studies have backed up these results.

Carnitine and Mental Energy

You'll recall that the ALA/ALC cocktail given to Dr. Ames's rats improved their memory power, enhancing their performance on maze tests. In further investigations, the scientists examined the brains of rats who had been given these supplements, and found:

- Less free radical damage to genetic material in the *hippocampus*, the part of the brain most affected by aging; damage was less in animals that got either ALA or ALC, but benefit was greatest in animals that got both.

- Hippocampal mitochondria were less damaged by aging in animals that got ALA, ALC, or both.

Research on the use of ALC in Alzheimer's disease hasn't conclusively shown it to be helpful at slowing cognitive decline—at least, not in any but the most mild cases of the disease.

Carnitine for . . . Sperm Fatigue?!

A study of 101 men found that the higher the concentration of L-carnitine in semen, the greater the number, motility, and percentage of "normal appearing" sperm. One study found that carnitine supplementation for three or four months significantly improves sperm motility.

Sperm Motility
The speed and dexterity with which sperm swim.

A study published in the journal *Urology* involved men aged sixty to seventy-four who had depressed mood, fatigue, and sexual dysfunction. They took either propionyl-L-carnitine plus acetyl-L-carnitine (2 grams a day of each) or testosterone. A third group got a placebo. After six months, both the testosterone and carnitine groups had similar results on tests of heart and sexual function. Depression was relieved by both therapies. Carnitine appeared to be better at enhancing the number of spontaneous erections a man experiences while asleep. Benefits of both testosterone and carnitine dissipated soon after either treatment was stopped.

Testosterone is somewhat riskier than carnitine.

Supplementation of that hormone has been linked with prostate problems, including cancer, and its use requires close physician supervision. For men in their "golden years" who feel like their spark is gone, a trial of carnitine might be worth a try.

Carnitine for Chronic Fatigue Syndrome and Multiple Sclerosis

In 1997, two researchers at the Chronic Fatigue Syndrome Center at the University of Chicago published their second study on carnitine and CFS, in the journal *Neuropsychobiology*. Research previous to this—including one in their own lab—had found low levels of carnitine and evidence of mitochondrial dysfunction in CFS patients. The lower the carnitine levels, the worse the CFS symptoms.

The University of Chicago team found that L-carnitine supplements yielded significant improvements in twelve of eighteen clinical parameters after eight weeks' treatment. It proved more effective than amantadine, a prescription medication used to treat fatigue in some CFS patients.

Patients with multiple sclerosis (MS) struggle against extreme fatigue, and amantadine has been found to help relieve this symptom. Amantadine has a long list of side effects that make it a less-than-ideal medicine, including insomnia, nausea, and dizziness. A study published in the *Journal of Neurological Science* in 2004 found that L-carnitine worked better than amantadine to relieve fatigue on one of the commonly used measuring scales of fatigue, the Fatigue Severity Scale.

> You'll find carnitine often billed as a weight-loss aid, but studies supporting this use aren't solid enough to support any claims that it helps shed pounds.

How to Use Carnitine

Carnitine is nontoxic, with mild side effects—diarrhea, increased appetite, and body rash—potentially appearing at 5 grams or more per day.

At this writing, the burning question of which form of carnitine to use has no firm answer. Studies of the simplest, least expensive form, L-carnitine, have shown promise, as have both the propionyl and acetyl forms of the nutrient. As it is, most of the research has involved the acetyl or L- forms of carnitine. I would recommend trying these forms first.

Try 500 to 1,000 milligrams a day for general improvements in energy and health; 2,000 to 3,000 milligrams (in divided doses) for fatigue, heart problems, infertility, or chronic fatigue syndrome. Take this supplement with a low-carb, high-protein dinner, along with your CoQ_{10} and alpha-lipoic acid. Oh, and don't forget to study up on the Macarena!

CHAPTER 6

QUICK ENERGY: RIBOSE AND CREATINE

Much of this book has been devoted to the use of nutrients for boosting energy in people who aren't in the best of health. The research on the supplements covered in the chapters up to this point has not demonstrated their usefulness as *ergogenic aids* or as *anabolic aids*. In this chapter and in the one following, we turn to supplements that are believed to work on one or both of these fronts.

Ergogenic Aids
Substances that can be used to improve athletic performance.

Modern athletes and bodybuilders use a lot of supplements. Many are always on the lookout for the next hot supplement that will help them perform better, put on more muscle, and beat the competition.

Anabolic Aids
Substances that help to build bigger muscles.

Two supplements appear to fit the bill particularly well when it comes to effectiveness and safety for athletes who need quick, intense bursts of energy for their workouts: *ribose* and *creatine*. Both supplements also show some promise in helping people who are less well move toward better energy and health.

Anaerobic versus Aerobic

Let's review the differences between sprint activity, which requires a big burst of ATP, *fast*, and is over quickly, and endurance activity, which requires a much lower-intensity effort for a longer period of time.

If you were in a race from here to the neighbor's house, how fast you ought to run has a lot to do with the distance you will be traveling. You'd be foolish to launch into a lung-busting sprint if the house is a mile away. If it's only twenty-five yards, you're sure to lose the race if you set off at a leisurely jog.

Sprint activity is anaerobic—it relies upon ATP production that happens so quickly that oxygen doesn't have time to get to the working muscles. Sprinting rapidly uses up energy stored in muscles as *glycogen*. Most of that energy is made through glycolysis, which you'll recall is less efficient than the Krebs cycle and oxidative phosphorylation. Lactic acid quickly accumulates in the working muscles, potentially leading to "the burn"—or, at the very least, to fatigue.

Glycogen
The storage form of glucose found in the liver and muscles.

Once you finish the sprint, muscle goes into recovery mode, and this process relies on the Krebs cycle and oxidative phosphorylation. That's why sprinters who are interviewed just after running at breakneck speed for less than ten seconds are huffing and puffing. They do this for some time after the event is over, moving oxygen to the muscles for aerobic metabolism, reducing lactic acid levels, and replenishing energy spent during the sprint.

In twenty-four to forty-eight hours following a bodybuilder's weight-training session—which is essentially a sprint workout with bursts of hard work interspersed with rest—changes take place in the muscle that make it bigger and stronger. Microscopic muscle damage is repaired, more strongly than before. The strengthening brought about by anaerobic activity happens not during the workout, but *between* workouts.

Aerobic activity is any physical work sustained longer than a couple of minutes, where your heart rate increases by twenty to forty beats per minute, you breathe heavily, and you break a sweat. Energy utilization is slow enough that the body can get oxygen to the muscles for efficient energy production. Walking, swimming, bicycling, dancing, and even light weight training (high reps, low weight) are all aerobic. In exercise science terms, aerobic exercise may be referred to as endurance exercise. Aerobic exercise capacity is dependent upon efficient energy production in the mitochondria, which in turn is dependent upon the ability of the lungs and heart to deliver enough oxygen to the muscles to prevent lactic acid buildup.

Ribose and creatine are primarily used to increase anaerobic power. If you are interested in aids for athletic endurance, look to Chapter 7, where we go into detail about adaptogenic herbs.

The Role of Ribose

DNA and RNA are the genetic "template" for new cells and for the synthesis of proteins. Proteins are an important building material for the construction of tissues, including muscle tissue. Ribose is a carbohydrate that creates the "backbone" of both DNA and RNA, as well as the vitamins B_2 and B_{12}. It also takes part in the metabolic process that produces ATP, the body's energy currency. Ribose exists in all living cells. Research evidence suggests that supplemental ribose helps to more rapidly regenerate ATP, speeding recovery from intense exercise.

In a Danish study, eight subjects did intensive sprint training for seven days. After the week-long training, they took three days off, during which they got either a ribose supplement or placebo three times per day. Muscle ATP levels were low at five and twenty-four hours following the last exercise session. At seventy-two hours, muscle ATP had returned to pretraining levels in the ribose group, but not in the placebo group.

In a study performed at the Applied Physiology Laboratory at Eastern Michigan University in Ypsilanti, Michigan, researchers evaluated the effects of ribose supplements on performance of sprint cycling tests in healthy subjects. Twice in one day, the subjects did six ten-second sprints, with sixty-second rest periods in between. After the second set of sprints, the subjects took 32 grams of ribose or a placebo—four doses of 8 grams each—over the next thirty-six hours, then returned to the lab to take the cycle test one more time. Then, after five days of no supplements or cycle testing, the whole thing was repeated again, switching the groups so that the initial ribose group got placebo and vice versa. Supplementation of ribose led to statistically significant increases in average power and peak power during and following the second sprint.

Ribose in Heart Disease and Fibromyalgia

Some evidence points to ribose as an aid in healing heart tissue damaged by lack of oxygen. Multiple animal studies have demonstrated that ribose improves the heart's energy metabolism and function following a heart attack.

Researchers at the University of Bonn in Germany assessed the effect of supplemental ribose on heart function and quality of life: in two three-week treatment periods, fifteen patients with coronary artery disease or heart failure were given either ribose or a placebo, with groups switched to the other treatment following the first three-week period. The hearts of patients on ribose had enhanced ability to fill with blood—an indication that damaged heart tissue was healing and regaining its strength. The ribose users also had significantly improved quality of life compared with the placebo group.

Coronary Artery Disease

Partly or completely clogged blood vessels to the heart.

Poor blood flow to any muscle results in ischemia. Ischemia compromises the rate at which ATP can be produced by limiting the availability of adenine nucleotides (the building blocks of ATP). Research suggests that ribose supplementation increases the availability of adenine nucleotides and ATP in previously oxygen-deprived tissues.

People with fibromyalgia tend to have severe chronic fatigue. Some try ribose in an effort to boost their energy. In one case study, a woman with fibromyalgia who added ribose to her supplement program experienced a noticeable reduction in symptoms.

Ribose: Summing Up

As ergogenic aids go, and for people suffering from heart disease, ribose appears to be worth a try. No side effects have been reported with its use.

To boost anaerobic power and aid in recovery after intense workouts, try 5 grams before and 5 grams immediately following exercise. For heart disease, try 5 grams two to three times a day. No harmful side effects have been reported.

Creatine: The Bodybuilder's Choice?

Creatine is a substance made in the liver from three amino acids: arginine, lysine, and methionine. It can be obtained through the diet in the form of meat and other animal products. Creatine is the most popular sports supplement in existence, and is used primarily by athletes whose workouts and competitions require quick bursts of power.

At the cellular level, creatine is transformed into a closely related substance called *phosphocrea-*

In order to help athletic performance, creatine *must be used in concert with an intelligently designed athletic training program,* specific to your sporting event.

tine. The first four to five seconds of a burst of intense activity are fueled by phosphocreatine, as creatine donates its phosphate group to turn ADP into ATP—serving as a reservoir of rapidly available energy.

Supplementation with creatine has been found to raise muscle levels of this fuel. In one well-designed study in competitive swimmers, it was found that creatine loading led to faster swimming times for up to four weeks after supplementation.

Other studies show that creatine supplementation, in healthy, athletic people, can:

- Increase muscular power over the course of several exercise sessions.

- Increase the maximal force an athlete can exert while jumping, sprinting, or cycling.

- Increase muscle size, primarily by pulling fluid into the muscle cells.

- Have slight benefit in reducing soreness following an exercise session.

- Help to buffer the buildup of lactic acid, enabling slightly harder training than could be achieved without heightened levels of carnitine.

Using Creatine

To use creatine as an ergogenic aid, add a loading dose of 20 grams per day for five to seven days, and stick with your training program. Thereafter, shift to a maintenance dose of two to five grams per day.

Be sure to drink plenty of water when using creatine to prevent dehydration. Side effects from high doses of creatine aren't common or serious, but can be bothersome: upset stomach, muscle cramps, and diarrhea have been reported. If you experience these side effects, stopping the supplement will quickly relieve them.

CHAPTER 7

RESERVE ENERGY: RHODIOLA AND GINSENG

Stressful life changes? Overworked? Tired all the time? Catching every "bug" that passes through your child's school? Prepping for a big exam? Want to win a marathon? Overwhelming scientific and historical evidence shows that adaptogens can help.

Adaptation describes the changes made in the body in response to changes in the environment. If you start a job that requires you to lift heavy objects all day, your muscles will get stronger and your endurance will improve as you adapt to the new level of activity. An adaptogen—usually, an herb—helps your body to adapt.

Adaptogens are most often used in an effort to fortify and strengthen the body and mind in the face of physical or mental stress. In doing so, many adaptogens have the overall effect of increasing physical and mental energy so that the body and mind can meet and overcome the challenges being faced. They boost stamina and immune function. Herbs classed as adaptogens have an overall normalizing effect; they help to relieve a wide variety of health problems by promoting balance in the body.

Current research—including some promising lab studies on cancer—has found that adaptogens may also help to *prevent* some common health problems, particularly those related to aging. The adage "an old dog can't learn new tricks" has some foundation in the physiology of aging: humans, as they age, lose at least some of their adaptability, and this causes more wear and tear on the body as it encounters stresses it's not able to adapt to.

An Herbal Link from Past to Present

Adaptogens have been in use throughout the world for millennia. Rhodiola and ginseng have been used since antiquity in Chinese medicine and eastern Europe. But it looks as though we may need the benefits of these herbs more than any of our predecessors did.

The pace of progress in modern civilization is breakneck, and the requirements for adaptation to that progress are considerable. Because our environments shift and change more quickly than ever before, it makes sense to use medicinal adaptogenic herbs—which are totally safe for most people, with the exception of those who are using multiple prescription drugs—to strengthen our ability to adapt to those changes.

How Adaptogens Work Their Wonders

With a stimulant, such as caffeine, you experience a burst of energy, followed by a slump that begs for further caffeination. Adaptogens take longer to "kick in," but once you have used them for a period of a few weeks, your body functions better and remains in a steadier balance.

Adaptogens are believed to work through a balance of "activating" and "deactivating" effects in the body:

1. *Activating effects:* where hormonal and other body communications systems are switched on by the herb, enhancing energy and improving the body's ability to use that energy.

2. *Deactivating effects:* where cellular communications are affected by adaptogens in ways that protect cells—and the whole organism—against overreacting to the factors switched on by the herb's activating effects.

Armenian researchers, in an article published in the journal *Phytomedicine*, call plant adaptogens "smooth pro-stressors," a term that encompasses both their energizing and calming effects. It's like the clear, energized feeling after a yoga session, instead of overstimulation and exhaustion after an all-out training session in a crowded gym.

When you look at adaptogenic effects in this light, you can see how a single herb, which contains a complex combination of plant chemicals and nutrients, could have an overall balancing effect on the body.

Rhodiola Overview

This herbal adaptogen comes from the root of a plant native to mountainous parts of the Arctic, Asia, and Europe. Rhodiola is also traditionally known as "golden root." Over two hundred species of this herb have been identified in the wild!

In a review of studies on this herb, published in the journal *Alternative Medicine Reviews* in 2001, author/researcher G. S. Kelly writes that rhodiola has been credited with "stimulating the nervous system, decreasing depression, enhancing work performance, eliminating fatigue, and preventing high altitude sickness" and that it also is believed to have "antidepressant, anticancer, cardioprotective, and central nervous system enhancement" properties. And Kelly cites research that indicates "great utility in asthenic conditions (decline in work performance, sleep difficulties, poor appetite, irritability, hypertension, headaches, and fatigue)."

Rhodiola's Active Constituents

Golden root contains a wide range of compounds with tried and true antioxidant activity, including p-tyrosol, caffeic acid, and proanthocyanidins. Other compounds in the plant are believed to influence levels and activity of neurotransmitters such as serotonin, norepinephrine, and dopamine.

Neuro-transmitters
Body chemicals that have enormous effects on mood and body functions.

Plant chemicals found in rhodiola also appear to have heart-protective properties, easing the effects of stress on heart cells. Rhodiola has also been found to buffer release of the hormone *cortisol* from the adrenal glands during times of stress. (Later in this chapter, you will learn that while cortisol is crucial for survival, too much is dangerous.)

Let's have a brief look at some of the most current studies on rhodiola, health, and energy levels:

- A 2004 study by the Russian government found that rhodiola rosea supplements reduced C-reactive protein in subjects' bodies—a sure sign of anti-inflammatory action. Following exhaustive exercise, subjects who took rhodiola had less muscle damage.

- Another study from Russia found that rhodiola root increased ATP content in the mitochondria of subjects' muscles, helping to regenerate it during workouts and during the recovery period.

- Belgian researchers found that in healthy, young volunteers, a single dose of rhodiola just before an endurance exercise test significantly improved their performance on that test.

- In a group of students, rhodiola extract yielded improvements in fitness, motor function, and well-being, with reduced need for sleep and improved stability of mood.

- Chinese researchers have published several studies showing that rhodiola extract reduces the biochemical effects of stress in rats subjected to loud noises.

- Several studies, many from Russian investigators, have found that rhodiola improves alertness and relieves mental fatigue in students (notably, medical students).

- Experimental studies in rats with hepatitis suggest that rhodiola has a liver-protective effect.

- Rhodiola was administered in an experimental model of ischemic stroke (caused by blockage in a brain blood vessel). Compared with a placebo, it slowed the development of physiological changes in the affected brain tissue: swelling, lactic acid accumulation, and free radical accumulation.

Rarely, those who take rhodiola experience insomnia or irritability.

Choose a *Rhodiola rosea* extract (the variety that has been most studied) standardized to 1 to 2 percent rosavin. Use 300 to 600 milligrams a day of the 1 percent extract or 180 to 300 milligrams a day of the 2 percent. Some extracts are standardized to 3.6 percent; if you choose this strength, take 100 to 170 milligrams per day. For general energy enhancement, begin taking it a few weeks before you expect to encounter increased stress, or before your endurance athletic event, and continue to use it until the stress or event has passed. You can also take three times this dose on a one-time basis to get pumped up for a stressful occasion or a competition.

If you use rhodiola or any adaptogen long-term, it's best to use it for a few weeks, then take a week or two off before starting again.

Any person using multiple prescription medications, particularly psychiatric drugs or the anticlotting drug warfarin, should confer with a physician and a pharmacist before adding rhodiola to their supplement plan.

Are Your Adrenals Exhausted?

The ginsengs are believed to work through balancing and tonifying effects on the interaction between the brain and the *endocrine* (hormonal) system—specifically, the adrenal glands, which are responsible for the production of a hormone called cortisol.

The adrenal glands sit atop the kidneys. They are divided into an inner layer, called the *medulla*, and an outer layer that wraps around it like a thick skin, called the *cortex.* In the medulla, *adrenaline* is made—the "fight-or-flight" hormone that is cranked out quickly in response to high stress, enabling the body to fight, flee, or take other high-energy action. Alterations in adrenaline production have been linked with symptoms of chronic fatigue syndrome.

The adrenal cortex makes two hormones that are vitally important for maintaining energy, and that are often found to be at low levels in people who lack energy: *cortisol* and *dehydroepiandrosterone* (DHEA). While DHEA levels naturally fall with aging, cortisol levels may actually rise with passing years. Cortisol is a slower-onset, longer-lasting fight-or-flight hormone that increases blood pressure, tamps down immunity, diverts blood flow from the internal organs and the thinking parts of the brain to the muscles, increases heart rate and respiratory rate, and generally prepares the body to either fight or flee.

People who are often under high stress, who eat too much sugar or drink too many caffeinated beverages (both of which elicit cortisol secretion), can over time become cortisol deficient. In essence, too-high demand on the adrenals depletes them. The result? Chronic fatigue. According to Jacob Teitelbaum, M.D., expert on CFS and author of the book *From Fatigued to Fantastic!*, about two-thirds of chronic fatigue patients appear to have underactive adrenal glands.

Symptoms Dr. Teitelbaum describes as indicative of adrenal exhaustion are fatigue, recurrent infections (particularly sore throat) that are hard to fight off, achiness, low blood sugar, low blood pressure (usually causes dizziness when going from sitting or lying down to standing), and tendency to "crash" during stressful periods rather than rising to meet the increased demands of life.

I've treated a lot of patients whose adrenals were depleted. Herbs and other supplements usually aren't enough to renew their energy. If you suspect your adrenals are exhausted, ask your doctor to test your morning cortisol, which needs to be done with a fasting blood sample drawn before 9:30 A.M., and a DHEA-S (the sulfated form of DHEA) test. The best, safest treatment for low output of adrenal hormones is *hydrocortisone* (Cortef), a drug version of cortisol that is identical to that made in the body (available by prescription); or an over-the-counter supplement called Isocort, a sheep's adrenal gland extract made by a company called Bezwecken that contains 1.5 to 2 milligrams of natural hydrocortisone per tablet; and DHEA, available over the counter as a supplement.

The usual dose of Cortef is one to three 5-milligram tablets per day, in divided doses, with the last dose taken at 4 P.M. or earlier. Work with your doctor to find the lowest dose that pulls you out of your slump. Isocort is taken twice daily, too.

DHEA shouldn't be used by people under forty if they are not shown to be deficient in lab tests. If you do require it and you are male, take 10 to 50 milligrams per day; if you're female, start with 10 to 25 milligrams every other day. Masculinizing side effects can occur in women, but they go away as soon as the DHEA is stopped.

Ginseng

If you were to go to the health food store to buy ginseng, you would likely encounter Asian (*Panax*) ginseng, sometimes referred to as Chinese ginseng, Panax ginseng, or Korean ginseng; American ginseng (*Panax quinquefolius*), which is thought to have milder effects; and Siberian ginseng (*Eleutherococcus senticosus*), which isn't really ginseng at all, but an entirely different plant so named because its effects on the body are similar to those of ginseng.

Here, we'll talk about Panax ginseng and Siberian ginseng. Both of these adaptogens have substantial support in scientific literature.

Panax Ginseng

Panax ginseng is a plant that grows well in parts of China, Russia, and Korea. Traditional Chinese medicine (TCM) practitioners have used its roots to treat fatigue and weakness for thousands of years. Ginseng's active ingredients are believed to be its *ginsenosides*. The best modern ginseng supplements are standardized for specific content of these plant chemicals.

Much of the scientific support for Panax ginseng as an ergogenic aid have more to do with mental endurance and performance than physical. A study of menopausal women found that sixteen weeks of ginseng supplementation improved their performance on a clinical test of well-being.

Some evidence suggests that ginseng could be useful for reducing blood sugars and boosting mood in diabetics. There is fairly solid evidence of positive effects on immunity, with increased antibody response to flu vaccination in one study and improved bacterial clearance in bronchitis patients on antibiotics plus ginseng.

A group of forty-five men with erectile dysfunction were given either Korean red ginseng (same as Panax ginseng) or placebo. The men on ginseng had improved desire and performance. And, finally, in a study of 4,364 people aged forty and older, cancer risk was more than halved in ginseng users.

High-stress lifestyles can lead to chronic oversecretion of cortisol, which over time can lead to hypertension, changes in insulin activity, carbohydrate cravings, and accumulation of belly fat. By modulating the production of this hormone, ginseng defuses these potentially harmful effects of stress on the body. In the case of adrenal exhaustion, ginseng is believed to support the endocrine system in its energy-enhancing processes.

On rare occasions, Panax ginseng users experience nausea, diarrhea, insomnia, euphoria, headaches, breast pain, unusual vaginal bleeding, or high or low blood pressure while using Panax ginseng. Using Panax with caffeine could raise blood pressure too high. Don't use Panax ginseng if you take warfarin (the herb can reduce the medicine's effectiveness) or the antidepressant drug phenelzine (brand name Nardil; can spur manic symptoms when used with this herb).

Use a Panax ginseng supplement standardized to 1.5 to 7 percent ginsenosides—some sources suggest that 4 percent is optimal. Standard doses range from 200 to 600 milligrams per day.

Siberian Ginseng (*Eleuthero*)

If you're seeking a boost in physical energy or endurance, Siberian ginseng—often called *Eleuthero*—appears to be a better choice than Panax ginseng.

Dr. I. I. Brekhman, the Russian scientist who first coined the term "adaptogen," did a lot of his research on the benefits of eleuthero, starting in 1959. (Long before that time, it had been used in traditional Chinese medicine to enhance energy.) He saw eleuthero used by people who lived in harsh climates and had to do a great deal of physical labor.

In studies on healthy subjects, eleuthero supplementation:

• Improved endurance and resistance to cold in competitive skiers.

• Improved speed of work in telegraph operators and accuracy of work in proofreaders.

- May help delay memory loss and deterioration of thinking ability in people with Alzheimer's disease, especially in its early stages.

- Reduced sick days in a population of factory workers by 40 percent, and reduced overall sickness in this population by 50 percent.

- Improved physical resistance to high-stress circumstances; in the original series of Russian studies performed in the 1960s, with adults aged nineteen to seventy-two who took Siberian ginseng had better tolerance for motion sickness, could perform more physical labor, and could better perform tasks requiring precision and speed despite noise, heat, high altitude, and lack of oxygen

- Improved color perception, hearing acuity, and mental and physical work capacity in overly hot or cold conditions or at high altitude

In subjects with heart disease, eleuthero reduces chest pain, blood pressure, and cholesterol levels, and improves mood. Diabetic subjects have been found to experience reductions in blood sugars. Hypertensives and hypotensives (people with blood pressure that's too low) may be able to normalize their blood pressure with eleuthero.

Research suggests that Siberian ginseng improves both female and male fertility; it particularly has an effect on sperm count. Menopausal women and those with difficult menstruation may be helped by the tonifying effects of eleuthero on uterine muscles.

TCM uses eleuthero to reinforce the body's qi, or vital energy. In modern medical terms, this translates to a tonifying effect on the adrenals. It appears to be especially valuable for people with chronic fatigue syndrome and fibromyalgia, a related syndrome that usually involves fatigue.

Seek an eleuthero supplement standardized to 0.8 percent eleutherosides. Take 100 to 200 milligrams three times a day to help cope with stress; for chronic fatigue or other fatiguing conditions, take 100 to 300 milligrams for 60–90 days, with a seven-day break before starting your next course of treatment. WholeHealthMD.com recommends rotating eleuthero and Panax with each other for male infertility: take eleuthero for three weeks (100 to 300 milligrams a day), then 100 to 250 milligrams a day of Panax ginseng for two weeks.

Don't use eleuthero if you have high blood pressure. Check with your doctor if you are on any prescription drugs to make sure you won't have adverse drug interactions.

CHAPTER 8

HIGH-ENERGY HABITS: EXERCISE AND STRESS MANAGEMENT

In this chapter, you won't get the usual extended litany of reasons why exercise is important. You won't hear all the arguments in favor of daily stress-management practices. Unless you've been living under a rock, you already know that both are important aspects of a healthy lifestyle, and one or both help prevent heart disease, cancer, osteoporosis, Alzheimer's disease, obesity, diabetes, arthritis, and virtually every other ill that strikes aging individuals.

In the bulk of this chapter, we're going to give you tools to incorporate these practices into your already busy life, in case you haven't done so already.

This having been said, here are a few arguments in favor of exercise and stress reduction that you might not have heard. These practices:

- Reduce cortisol levels in the body.

- Increase day-to-day energy when done on a regular schedule.

- Have a tonifying effect on the nervous system that leads to reduced heart rate and blood pressure and improved mood.

- Amp up the body's production of the antioxidants it can make on its own.

- Aid in the body's ability to handle stressful situations without excessive "fight-or-flight" reactions.

- Improve immune-system function, enhancing the body's ability to fight off infections.

The Basics of an Energizing Exercise Program

When we exercise, we rev our cellular engines—running them through their paces, increasing energy demands on them in a controlled fashion. Doing so on a regular basis increases their endurance and work capacity. The circulatory system, the respiratory system, and the muscles all become more efficient. You have more energy to spare. There's a twinkle in your eye.

On the other hand, the person who *overexercises* will have diminishing returns. It's a common misconception that the athlete who puts enormous physical demands on his or her body is healthier than the person who exercises moderately. Hard athletic training can put undue stress on the body, reducing immunity and adding up to fatigue and injury. The same can happen for a person who is engaging in an intense workout program in an effort to lose weight.

If you are a recreational athlete or striving to lose a lot of weight with the help of a hard workout program, enlist the services of a qualified trainer or coach who can help you do enough, but not too much.

To design a moderate and energy-enhancing program, you'll need to do both cardiovascular and strengthening exercises. These two types of exercise will, over time, lead to drastically different but complementary changes in your body's ability to make and utilize energy.

Cardiovascular Workouts

This kind of exercise is often referred to as *aerobic*. Any activity that gets the major muscle groups of the body moving steadily for fifteen minutes or more, at an intensity that increases heart rate and breathing rate and brings on a sweat (if it's warm enough), is an aerobic activity. Walking is great; all you need is a good pair of shoes. Cycling, swimming, tennis, water aerobics, dancing, gardening, rock climbing, shooting hoops, ballet class, martial arts, housework, stair climbing, circuit training—the options are vast.

> **Circuit Training**
> *Circuit training consists of lifting light weights for 15–20 repetitions, while rotating around to stations that target various muscle groups.*

The most important aspect of aerobic activity is *consistency*—doing it at least three times a week, preferably every day. To foster this consistency, stop thinking of exercise as something you do in special clothes in a noisy gym for an hour, when you can get over there. You don't need to go to a gym, and you don't need to exercise for an hour straight to benefit. Recent research shows that several short sessions of activity throughout the day is just as health-enriching an approach—and it's an approach that may be better for promoting an even stream of mental and physical energy throughout the day.

Park at the far end of parking lots; walk to lunch if you can instead of driving; take the stairs instead of the elevator. If you have a desk job, try sitting on a large Thera-Ball instead of an office chair—this will keep your muscles active as you sit. Put an hourly reminder in your computer to take a five-minute walk and stretch your body. When you watch TV, sit on an exercycle or do some squats, stomach crunches, or other calisthenic-type exercises instead of sitting on the couch.

Don't stop doing longer, more intense workouts if you enjoy them. If that approach works for you, that's great, and you are reaping benefits too. Either way, it's about finding something that you can maintain long term.

Strength Training

Strength training entails pitting muscles against resistance to increase their strength. As strength increases, we increase the resistance. Weight training is the most common—but by no means the only—form of strength training (which is also known as resistance training).

In recent years, the fitness world has emphasized strength training as a way to total fitness. We were told that by adding muscle, we would then burn extra fat, even when we were at rest. Current wisdom contradicts this approach. A couple of pounds of extra muscle doesn't burn enough extra calories to have a significant impact on weight loss. A lot of overweight people already have big muscles, which they need to carry around all that extra weight. They need to eat fewer calories and do cardiovascular exercise to drop excess pounds.

A resistance training program can be done with hand weights or other equipment at home, or at the gym. Many gyms offer weight training classes. Some yoga classes—usually termed "power yoga" or "flow yoga"—offer benefits similar to resistance training. So, too, do martial arts and ballet or jazz dance classes. Thera-ball exercise programs are popular these days, as is Pilates, a form of physical training originally designed for ballet dancers. In the Resources section, you can find recommendations for books and videos to get you started with a home program. If you prefer the gym, talk with a trainer about setting you up with an effective, time-efficient program.

Stress Reduction: Yoga, Tai Chi, Chi Kung, and Other "Enlightened Exercise"

"Stress reduction" may actually not be the best term for what I am about to discuss. A better term is "reduction of the negative physical and psychological impact of stress." Our goal isn't to make stress go away, but to learn how to better handle it. This is where yoga, tai chi, and chi kung—what health writer Virginia Hopkins has called "enlightened exercise"—come into the big picture of your overall energy.

We call these practices "enlightened" because they embrace both the spiritual and the physical. You can practice them simply as exercises, but you get more out of them if you approach them as spiritual practices. Extensive research shows that people who follow a spiritual path are, overall, healthier and longer-lived than people who do not.

The spiritual modes of thought in yoga, tai chi, or chi kung do not conflict with more Western religious traditions; in fact, they can be strongly complementary to those traditions.

Enlightened exercise has two important effects on the body:

1. It trains the "fight-or-flight" hormonal and cardiovascular systems of the body to react less joltingly in the face of stress. For example, if you've been practicing yoga for a few months, and you get into a stressful argument with a co-worker, you will likely have cultivated the ability to breathe deeply and relax your body out of fight-or-flight mode. This helps you remain intelligent and balanced in the face of stress.

2. It trains the mind and body together in moving the body's vital energy around to where it is most needed. In tai chi and chi kung, both developed as adjuncts to traditional Chinese healing practices, the exerciser uses his mind to direct energy along pathways in the body (meridians) in ways that increase energy and defuse stress.

Yoga

If you think yoga is only for people who can wrap their legs around the back of their head, you are in for a pleasant surprise.

A yoga session is comprised of a series of poses,

most of them hundreds of years old. Most were originally designed with a specific healing or health-promoting purpose. The poses tone and stretch the muscles and improve balance, posture, and coordination. In some yoga classes, poses are threaded together with movements that exercise the cardiovascular system. Yoga also usually involves deep, measured breathing in time with the poses, and periods of quiet meditation.

If you are interested in trying yoga, seek out a beginner's class. A good teacher will be hands-on, guiding and coaching you into the poses, telling you how the energy moves through and out of your body when you are doing it right. Once you have learned how to do the poses properly, you can practice yoga at home. A fifteen-minute yoga session in the morning can give you serene, balanced energy throughout the day.

Yoga can be your resistance training workout, too. Many of the poses and movements of yoga involve strengthening of the leg, buttock, back, abdominal, and upper-body muscles.

Tai Chi

The word "chi" describes the life force that moves around within the body. With tai chi practice, we learn to mold and move that chi in ways that promote greater health and energy.

Tai chi is an excellent practice for elderly or arthritic individuals; it is gentle, relaxing, and rejuvenating, and supports better posture and alignment. Professional instruction is the best way to begin a tai chi practice. While some yoga poses can be dangerous if practiced without proper instruction, tai chi is safe to try on your own with videos or DVDs.

Chi Kung (Qigong)

Tai chi is one form of chi kung—a phonetic spelling of *qigong*. This ancient Chinese movement art involves breath, physical postures, and the focused movement of energy within the body.

Chi kung is about cultivating energy in specific ways to maintain and improve health and increase vitality. It can be used to increase energy, or to reduce or store energy away. Widely recommended by alternative healthcare practitioners, chi kung has been found in medical research to have positive effects on parameters of cardiorespiratory, digestive, and immune system health. It improves balance and is said to encourage a positive outlook.

Anyone can learn and practice chi kung, including children and the very old, the well and the very infirm. You should be able to find an instructor near you either in the phone book or by calling acupuncturists or schools that teach martial arts. There is also a National Qigong Association (www.nqa.org) that maintains a list of instructors. Or, try learning from a video or book (see the Resources section for recommendations).

Other Ways to Manage Stress

Even yogis and tai chi masters encounter stresses they need extra help to handle. Here are a few other techniques you can use to manage day-to-day stress:

Relaxation

This simple technique can be used once a day for five to thirty minutes to defuse the effects of stress on the body. Set a timer (without a jolting alarm) or put on a soothing piece of music so that you can relax until the session is over. Sit comfortably, close your eyes, and allow your muscles to relax. Let your breath deepen naturally, falling into a regular pattern. With each exhalation, repeat a word: try "relax" or "release," or a word with religious meaning to you; or, use the word "om" (ohhhhhm) commonly used in meditation practices.

Progressive Muscle Relaxation (PMR)

Sometimes, we're so tense that we can't even identify which muscles are tight. This is where Progressive Muscle Relaxation (PMR) is useful.

Sit or lie down with your feet slightly elevated. Tense the muscles in your face, clenching your teeth; hold it for five to ten seconds, then release, exhaling. Do the same with the muscles of the back of the head and neck; then, the shoulders; then the chest; then the arms and hands. Work your way from the top of your head to your toes. Allow the body parts to shed tension and feel warm and heavy as they relax.

Visualization

In the midst of a high-stress moment, imagine a place that is beautiful and restful: a windswept beach, a scenic mountaintop, a serene meditation room: your imagination is the only limit to the places you can take this "mini-vacation." Engage every sense. How does it smell? What sounds do you hear? What do you taste? Stay there for five to ten minutes, if possible, before returning to the present.

Focused Breathing

When your energy is going into a fight-or-flight stress response, your breaths get short and quick. Many people get into the habit of this kind of shallow breathing, and never take a really deep and cleansing breath unless they're asleep! Breath is a great tool for increasing overall energy in the body. Start deepening your own breath whenever you think of it. As you sit in a chair, allow your breaths to become fuller and deeper, expanding your abdomen, chest, and upper back with each inhale. Lie on the floor on your back and breathe deeply for a few minutes when tensions run high.

Other techniques to try: journaling, learning to

say "no" to commitments that are likely to over-whelm you, improving time management, engaging in social interaction, becoming a member of a community (church, interest or hobby group, arts group, charity), spending time in nature, having a massage or other bodywork, or counseling (particularly if your relationship with significant others or family members are a major source of intractable stress). Pets can also be a great source of relaxation.

When stress gets the better of you, your energy is drained into worry and anger. Most of us can't afford this kind of energy drain. Taking steps to improve one's ability to reserve energy in times of stress may not seem all that important in the daily grind, but it can make an enormous difference in your energy level and quality of life.

CONCLUSION

In high-school physics class, we learn that energy is *the capacity to do work or overcome resistance.* Types of energy include mechanical energy; thermal (heat) energy; and chemical, electrical, potential, and kinetic energies. You probably recall the first law of thermodynamics, also known as the law of conservation of energy: while energy can be transferred from one system to another, and can take many forms, it cannot be created or destroyed.

The energy that causes heat to radiate from a fire is the same energy that powers the contraction and relaxation of the muscle cells that make up a beating heart. The energy that makes your computer work is the same energy that crackles around in your brain cells while you read this book. It's just changing form.

Now you know that many factors affect your mental and physical experience of energy. It begins at the cellular level, where the mitochondria turn carbohydrates and fats into ATP through complex biochemical reactions—reactions that require the participation of many nutrients. Those energy-producing cells are what make your organs—the heart, the brain, the liver—that are constantly at work maintaining you as a working, functioning, breathing, sentient human being.

Alongside a healthful diet, you can use scientifically supported, safe supplemental nutrients to ensure that your cells have all the cogs, wheels, and sparks required for excellent and efficient energy production. This translates into a sense of increased vim and vigor in you. You're better able to weather life's storms—and to celebrate life's gifts.

Whether you are chronically fatigued and searching for relief or just looking for a little boost in your strength or endurance, energy nutrients can help you get where you want to go. I hope this User's Guide has helped you to learn which could be most useful for you.

SELECTED
REFERENCES

Arivazhagan P., Ramanathan K., and Panneerselvam C., "Effect of DL-alpha-lipoic acid on mitochondrial enzymes in aged rats," *Chemico-Biological Interactions* 2001 Nov 28;138(2):189–198.

Berardi J. M. and Ziegenfuss T. N., "Effects of ribose supplementation on repeated sprint performance in men," *Journal of Strength Conditioning Research* 2003 Feb;17(1):47–52.

Cavallini G., Caracciolo S., Vitali G., et al., "Carnitine versus androgen administration in the treatment of sexual dysfunction, depressed mood, and fatigue associated with aging," *Urology* 2004 Apr;63(4): 641–646.

Darbinyan V., Kteyan A., Panossian A., et al., "Rhodiola rosea in stress induced fatigue—a double-blind cross-over study of a standardized extract SHR-5 with a repeated low-dose regimen on the mental performance of healthy physicians during night duty," *Phytomedicine* 2000 Oct;7(5):365–371.

Golomb B.A., Criqui M.H., White H.L., et al., "Conceptual foundation of the UCSD Statin Study: A randomized controlled trial assessing the impact of statins on cognition, behavior and biochemistry," *Archives of Internal Medicine* 2004 Jan 26:164(2): 153–162.

Hagen T. M., Ingersoll R.T., Lykkesfeldt J., et al., "(R)-α-lipoic acid-supplemented old rats have improved mitochondrial function, decreased oxidative damage, and increased metabolic rate," *Federation of American Societies for Experimental Biology Journal (FASEB J)* 1999; http://www.fasebj.org/cgi/content/abstract/13/2/411.

Kelly G. S., "Rhodiola rosea: A possible plant adaptogen," *Alternative Medicine Reviews* 2001 Jun;6(3): 293–302.

Kiefer, David, M. D., and Traci Pantuso, B. S., "Panax ginseng," *American Family Physician* 2003 Oct 15; 68(8).

Liu J., Head E., Kuratsune H., et al., "Memory loss in old rats is associated with brain mitochondrial decay and RNA/DNA oxidation: Partial reversal by feeding acetyl-L-carnitine and/or R-alpha-lipoic acid," *Proceedings of the National Academy of Sciences USA* 2002; 99(4):2356–2361.

No authors listed, "Rejuvenation? Acetyl-L-carnitine and alpha-lipoic acid: Juvenon," http://nootropics. com/acetylcarnitine/rejuvenation.html.

Omran H., Illien S., MacCarter D., et al., "D-ribose improves diastolic function and quality of life in congestive heart failure patients: A prospective feasibility study," *European Journal of Heart Failure* 2003 Oct;5(5):615–619.

Panossian A., Wikman G., and Wagner H., "Plant adaptogens. III. Earlier and more recent aspects and concepts on their mode of action," *Phytomedicine* 1999 Oct;6(4):287–300.

Suh J. H., Shigeno E. T., Morrow J. D., et al., "Oxidative stress in the aging rat heart is reversed by dietary supplementation with (R)-alpha-lipoic acid," *Federation of American Societies for Experimental Biology Journal (FASEB J)* 2001 Mar;15(3):700–706.

Zhu B., Sun Y. M., Yun X., et al., "Resistance imparted by traditional Chinese medicines to the acute change of glutamic pyruvic transaminase, alkaline phosphatase and creatine kinase activities in rat blood caused by noise," *Bioscience, Biotechnology and Biochemistry* 2004 May;68(5):1160–1163.

OTHER BOOKS AND RESOURCES

Books

Feed Your Genes Right, by Jack Challem (John Wiley & Sons, 2005).

From Fatigued To Fantastic!: A Proven Program to Regain Vibrant Health, Based on a New Scientific Study Showing Effective Treatment for Chronic Fatigue and Fibromyalgia, by Jacob Teitelbaum, M.D. (Avery Books, 2001).

Full Catastrophe Living: Using the Wisdom of Your Body and Mind to Face Stress, Pain, and Illness, by Jon Kabat-Zinn, M.D. (Delta, 1990).

Men's Health Home Workout Bible: A Do-It-Yourself Guide to Burning Fat and Building Muscle, by Lou Schuler and Michael Mejia (Rodale Books, 2002).

Opening the Energy Gates of Your Body: The Tao of Energy Enhancement, by Bruce Kumar Frantzis (North Atlantic Books, 1993).

Strength Training for Women, by Joan Pagano (DK Adult, 2004).

The Complete Idiot's Guide to Tai Chi & Qigong, by Bill Douglas (Alpha, 2002).

The Low GI Diet Revolution, by Jennie Brand-Miller, Kaye Foster-Powell, and Joanna MacMillan-Price (Marlowe & Co., 2005).

The Raw Food Detox Diet, by Natalie Rose (Regan Books, 2005).

Weight Training for Dummies, by Liz Neporent and Suzanne Schlossberg (For Dummies Publishers, 2000).

Yoga: The Spirit and Practice of Moving into Stillness, by Erich Schiffman (Pocket Books, 1996).

DVDs and Videos

Pilates Workout for Dummies, with Michelle Doizos (Anchor Bay Entertainment, 2001).

Relaxation and Breathing for Meditation, with Rodney Yee (Gaiam Americas, 2003).

A.M. and P.M. Yoga for Beginners, with Rodney Yee (Living Arts, 2002).

On the Ball: Pilates Workout for Beginners with Lizbeth Garcia (Goldhil Home Media I, 2003).

Balance Ball for Beginners (Living Arts, 2002).

Magazines

GreatLife Magazine
Consumer magazine with articles on vitamins, minerals, herbs, and foods.
Available for free at many health and natural food stores.

Let's Live Magazine
Consumer magazine with emphasis on the health benefits of vitamins, minerals, and herbs.
Customer service:
1-800-676-4333
P.O. Box 74908
Los Angeles, CA 90004
Subscriptions: 12 issues per year, $19.95 in the U.S.; $31.95 outside the U.S.

Physical Magazine
Magazine oriented to body builders and other serious athletes.
Customer service:
1-800-676-4333
P.O. Box 74908
Los Angeles, CA 90004
Subscriptions: 12 issues per year, $19.95 in the U.S.; $31.95 outside the U.S.

The Nutrition Reporter™ newsletter

Monthly newsletter that summarizes recent medical research on vitamins, minerals, and herbs.

Customer service:

P.O. Box 30246

Tucson, AZ 85751-0246

e-mail: jack@thenutritionreporter.com

www.nutritionreporter.com

Subscriptions: $26 per year (12 issues) in the U.S.; $32 U.S. or $48 CNC for Canada; $38 for other countries

INDEX

Printed in the USA
CPSIA information can be obtained
at www.ICGtesting.com
JSHW051956150824
68134JS00050B/55